How to Read a Paper

The basics of evidence-based medicine

THIRD EDITION

In November 1995, my friend Ruth Holland, book reviews editor of the *British Medical Journal*, suggested that I write a book to demystify the important but often inaccessible subject of evidence-based medicine. She provided invaluable comments on earlier drafts of the manuscript, but was tragically killed in a train crash on 8 August 1996. This book is dedicated to her memory.

How to Read a Paper

The basics of evidence-based medicine

THIRD EDITION

Trisha Greenhalgh

Department of Primary Care and Population Sciences
University College London Medical School
Highgate Hill
London

Blackwell
Publishing

© BMJ Books 1997, 2001
© 2006 by Blackwell Publishing Ltd
BMJ Books is an imprint of the BMJ Publishing Group Limited, used under licence

Blackwell Publishing, Inc., 350 Main Street, Malden, Massachusetts 02148-5020, USA
Blackwell Publishing Ltd, 9600 Garsington Road, Oxford OX4 2DQ, UK
Blackwell Publishing Asia Pty Ltd, 550 Swanston Street, Carlton, Victoria 3053, Australia

The right of the Author to be identified as the Author of this Work has been asserted in
accordance with the Copyright, Designs and Patents Act 1988.

First published 1997   Second edition 2001
Second impression 1997   Second impression 2001
Third impression 1998   Third impression 2002
Fourth impression 1998   Fourth impression 2002
Fifth impression 1999   Fifth impression 2003
Sixth impression 2000   Sixth impression 2003
Seventh impression 2000   Seventh impression 2004
                              Reprinted 2004
                              Third edition 2006

2   2006

ISBN-13: 978-1-4051-3976-2
ISBN-10: 1-4051-3976-5

A catalogue record for this title is available from the British Library and the
Library of Congress

Set in 9.5/12pt Minion by Newgen Imaging Systems (P) Ltd, Chennai, India
Printed and bound by TJ International, Padstow, UK

Commissioning Editor: Mary Banks
Editorial Assistant: Ariel Vernon
Development Editor: Nick Morgan
Production Controller: Debbie Wyer

For further information on Blackwell Publishing, visit our website:
http://www.blackwellpublishing.com

The publisher's policy is to use permanent paper from mills that operate a sustainable
forestry policy, and which has been manufactured from pulp processed using acid-free and
elementary chlorine-free practices. Furthermore, the publisher ensures that the text paper
and cover board used have met acceptable environmental accreditation standards.

Contents

Foreword to the First Edition
by Professor Sir David Weatherall

Not surprisingly, the wide publicity given to what is now called 'evidence-based medicine' has been greeted with mixed reactions by those who are involved in the provision of patient care. The bulk of the medical profession appears to be slightly hurt by the concept, suggesting as it does that until recently all medical practice was what Lewis Thomas has described as a frivolous and irresponsible kind of human experimentation, based on nothing but trial and error, and usually resulting in precisely that sequence. On the other hand, politicians and those who administrate our health services have greeted the notion with enormous glee. They had suspected all along that doctors were totally uncritical and now they had it on paper. Evidence-based medicine came as a gift from the gods because, at least as they perceived it, its implied efficiency must inevitably result in cost saving.

The concept of controlled clinical trials and evidence-based medicine is not new however. It is recorded that Frederick II, Emperor of the Romans and King of Sicily and Jerusalem, who lived from 1192 to 1250 AD, and who was interested in the effects of exercise on digestion, took two knights and gave them identical meals. One was then sent out hunting and the other ordered to bed. At the end of several hours he killed both and examined the contents of their alimentary canals; digestion had proceeded further in the stomach of the sleeping knight. In the seventeenth century Jan Baptista van Helmont, a physician and philosopher, became sceptical of the practice of bloodletting. Hence he proposed what was almost certainly the first clinical trial involving large numbers, randomisation and statistical analysis. This involved taking 200–500 poor people, dividing them into two groups by casting lots, and protecting one from phlebotomy while allowing the other to be treated with as much bloodletting as his colleagues thought appropriate. The number of funerals in each group would be used to assess the efficacy of bloodletting. History does not record why this splendid experiment was never carried out.

If modern scientific medicine can be said to have had a beginning it was in Paris in the mid-nineteenth century and where it had its roots in the work and teachings of Pierre Charles Alexandre Louis. Louis introduced statistical analysis to the evaluation of medical treatment and, incidentally, showed that bloodletting was a valueless form of treatment, though this did not change the habits of the physicians of the time, or for many years to come. Despite this pioneering work few clinicians on either side of the Atlantic urged that trials of clinical outcome should be adopted, although the principles of numerically based experimental design were enunciated in the 1920s by the geneticist Ronald Fisher. The field only started to make a major impact on clinical practice after the Second World War following the seminal work of Sir Austin Bradford Hill and the British epidemiologists who followed him, notably Richard Doll and Archie Cochrane.

But although the idea of evidence-based medicine is not new, modern disciples like David Sackett and his colleagues are doing a great service to clinical practice, not just by popularising the idea but by bringing home to clinicians the notion that it is not a dry academic subject but more a way of thinking that should permeate every aspect of medical practice. While much of it is based on mega-trials and meta-analyses it should also be used to influence almost everything that a doctor does. After all, the medical profession has been brain-washed for years by examiners in medical schools and Royal Colleges to believe that there is only one way of examining a patient. Our bedside rituals could do with as much critical evaluation as our operations and drug regimes; the same goes for almost every aspect of doctoring.

As clinical practice becomes busier, and time for reading and reflection becomes even more precious, the ability effectively to peruse the medical literature and, in the future, to become familiar with a knowledge of best practice from modern communication systems, will be essential skills for doctors. In this lively book, Trisha Greenhalgh provides an excellent approach to how to make best use of medical literature and the benefits of evidence-based medicine. It should have equal appeal for first-year medical students and grey-haired consultants, and deserves to be read widely.

With increasing years the privilege of being invited to write a foreword to a book by one's ex-students becomes less of a rarity. Trisha Greenhalgh was the kind of medical student who never let her teachers get away with a loose thought and this inquiring attitude seems to have flowered over the years; this is a splendid and timely book and I wish it all the success it deserves. After all, the concept of evidence-based medicine is nothing more than the state of mind that every clinical teacher hopes to develop in their students; Dr Greenhalgh's sceptical but constructive approach to medical literature suggests that such a happy outcome is possible at least once in the lifetime of a professor of medicine.

D.J. Weatherall
Oxford, September 1996

Preface to the Third Edition

When I wrote this book in 1996, evidence-based medicine was a bit of an unknown quantity. A handful of academics (including me) were already enthusiastic and had begun running 'training the trainers' courses to disseminate what we saw as a highly logical and systematic approach to clinical practice. Others – certainly the majority of clinicians – were convinced that this was a passing fad that was of limited importance and would never catch on. I wrote *How to Read a Paper* for two reasons. First, students on my own courses were asking for a simple introduction to the principles presented in what was then known as 'Dave Sackett's big red book' (Sackett DL, Haynes RB, Guyatt GH, Tugwell P. *Clinical epidemiology – a basic science for clinical medicine*, London: Little, Brown & Co., 1991) – an outstanding and inspirational volume that was already in its fourth reprint, but which some novices apparently found a hard read. Second, it was clear to me that many of the critics of evidence-based medicine didn't really understand what they were dismissing – and that until they did, serious debate on the political, ideological and pedagogical place of evidence-based medicine as a discipline could not begin.

I am of course delighted that *How to read a paper* has become a standard reader in many medical and nursing schools, and that it has so far been translated into French, German, Italian, Spanish, Chinese, Polish, Japanese and Russian. I am also delighted that what was so recently a fringe subject in academia has been well and truly mainstreamed in clinical service. In the United Kingdom, for example, it is now a contractual requirement for all doctors, nurses and pharmacists to practise (and for managers to manage) according to best research evidence.

In the 10 years since the first edition of this book was published, evidence-based medicine has waxed and waned in popularity. Some 500 textbooks and 15,000 journal articles now offer different angles on the 'basics of EBM' covered briefly in the chapters that follow. An increasing number of these sources point out genuine limitations of evidence-based medicine in certain contexts. Others look at evidence-based medicine as a social movement – a 'bandwagon' that took off at a particular time (the 1990s) and place (North America) and spread dramatically quickly with all sorts of knock-on effects for particular interest groups.

When preparing this third edition, I was advised by my publisher not to change too much, since there is clearly still room on the bookshelves for a no-frills introductory text. Many of the chapters are essentially unchanged apart from adding illustrations and updating the reference lists. Some chapters – notably those on searching, qualitative research, systematic review and implementing evidence-based practice – have been fundamentally revised because the fields have moved on significantly since the previous edition. I've also added a completely new chapter on questionnaire research. As ever, I'd welcome any feedback that will help make the text more accurate, readable and practical.

Trisha Greenhalgh
July 2005

Preface to the First Edition: do you need to read this book?

This book is intended for anyone, whether medically qualified or not, who wishes to find their way into the medical literature, assess the scientific validity and practical relevance of the articles they find and, where appropriate, put the results into practice. These skills constitute the basics of evidence-based medicine.

I hope this book will help you to read and interpret medical papers better. I hope, in addition, to convey a further message, which is this. Many of the descriptions given by cynics of what evidence-based medicine is (the glorification of things that can be measured without regard for the usefulness or accuracy of what is measured, the uncritical acceptance of published numerical data, the preparation of all-encompassing guidelines by self-appointed 'experts' who are out of touch with real medicine, the debasement of clinical freedom through the imposition of rigid and dogmatic clinical protocols and the over-reliance on simplistic, inappropriate and often incorrect economic analyses) are actually criticisms of what the evidence-based medicine movement is fighting *against*, rather than of what it represents.

Do not, however, think of me as an evangelist for the gospel according to evidence-based medicine. I believe that the science of finding, evaluating and implementing the results of medical research can, and often does, make patient care more objective, more logical and more cost-effective. If I didn't believe that, I wouldn't spend so much of my time teaching it and trying, as a general practitioner, to practise it. Nevertheless, I believe that when applied in a vacuum (i.e. in the absence of common sense and without regard to the individual circumstances and priorities of the person being offered treatment or to the complex nature of clinical practice and policy making), 'evidence-based' decision making is a reductionist process with a real potential for harm.

Finally, you should note that I am neither an epidemiologist nor a statistician, but a person who reads papers and who has developed a pragmatic (and at times unconventional) system for testing their merits. If you wish to pursue the epidemiological or statistical themes covered in this book, I would encourage you to move on to a more definitive text, references for which you will find at the end of each chapter.

Trisha Greenhalgh
November 1996

Acknowledgements

I am not by any standards an expert on all of the subjects covered in this book (in particular, I am very bad at sums), and I am grateful to the people listed below for help along the way. I am, however, the final author of every chapter, and responsibility for any inaccuracies is mine alone.

1 To Professor Sir Andy Haines and Professor Dave Sackett who introduced me to the subject of evidence-based medicine and encouraged me to write about it.

2 To Dr Anna Donald, who broadened my outlook through valuable discussions on the implications and uncertainties of this evolving discipline.

3 To Jeanette Buckingham, Librarian, John W. Scott Health Sciences Library, University of Alberta, Canada, for invaluable input to Chapter 2.

4 To numerous expert advisers and proofreaders of this edition. In addition, this edition builds on the input of people who advised me on previous editions of this book, whose names are listed in full in the earlier editions.

5 To the many people, too numerous to mention individually, who took time to write in and point out both typographical and factual errors in the first and second editions. As a result of their contributions, I have learnt a great deal (especially about statistics) and the book has been improved in many ways. Some of the earliest critics of *How to read a paper* have subsequently worked with me on my teaching courses in evidence-based practice; several have co-authored other papers or book chapters with me, and one or two have become personal friends.

6 To various colleagues, named in the different chapters, who gave permission for me to reproduce figures and tables. Box 10.2 of Chapter 10, reproduced from Tony Hope and colleagues' book *Medical ethics and law; the core curriculum*, is based on data provided by Dr A. Briggs and Professor A. Gray, Department of Public Health, University of Oxford.

Thanks also to my family for sparing me the time and space to finish this book.

Chapter 1 **Why read papers at all?**

1.1 Does 'evidence-based medicine' simply mean 'reading papers in medical journals'?

Evidence-based medicine (EBM) is much more than just reading papers. According to the most widely quoted definition, it is 'the conscientious, explicit and judicious use of current best evidence in making decisions about the care of individual patients'.[1] I find this definition very useful but it misses out what for me is a very important aspect of the subject – that is, the use of mathematics. Even if you know almost nothing about evidence-based medicine you know it talks a lot about numbers and ratios! Anna Donald and I decided to be upfront about this in our own teaching, and proposed this alternative definition:

> Evidence-based medicine is the use of mathematical estimates of the risk of benefit and harm, derived from high-quality research on population samples, to inform clinical decision making in the diagnosis, investigation or management of individual patients.

The defining feature of evidence-based medicine, then, is the use of figures derived from research on *populations* to inform decisions about *individuals*. This, of course, begs the question 'What is research'? – for which a reasonably accurate answer might be 'Focused, systematic enquiry aimed at generating new knowledge'. In later chapters, I explain how this definition can help you distinguish genuine research (which should inform your practice) from the poor-quality endeavours of well-meaning amateurs (which you should politely ignore).

If you follow an evidence-based approach to clinical decision making, all sorts of issues relating to your patients (or, if you work in public health medicine, issues relating to groups of patients) will prompt you to ask questions about scientific evidence, seek answers to those questions in a systematic way and alter your practice accordingly.

You might ask questions about a patient's symptoms ('e.g. in a 34-year-old man with left-sided chest pain, what is the probability that there is a serious heart problem, and if there is, will it show up on a resting ECG?'), about physical or diagnostic signs ('e.g. in an otherwise uncomplicated childbirth, does the presence of meconium [indicating fetal bowel movement] in the amniotic fluid indicate significant deterioration in the physiological state of the fetus?'), about the prognosis of an illness ('e.g. if a previously well 2 year old has a short fit associated with a high temperature, what is the chance that she will subsequently develop epilepsy?'), about therapy ('e.g. in patients with an acute myocardial infarction [heart attack], are the risks associated with thrombolytic drugs [clotbusters] outweighed by the benefits, whatever the patient's age, sex and ethnic origin?'), about cost-effectiveness ('e.g. in order to reduce the suicide rate in a health district, is it better to employ more consultant psychiatrists, more community psychiatric nurses or more counselors?'), about patients' preferences ('e.g. in women attending a male doctor for a vaginal examination, what proportion would like to be offered a chaperone?') and about a host of other aspects of health and health services.

Professor Dave Sackett, in the opening editorial of the very first issue of the journal *Evidence-Based Medicine*, summarised the essential steps in the emerging science of evidence-based medicine:[2]

1 to convert our information needs into answerable questions (i.e. to formulate the problem);
2 to track down, with maximum efficiency, the best evidence with which to answer these questions – which may come from the clinical examination, the diagnostic laboratory, the published literature or other sources;
3 to appraise the evidence critically (i.e. weigh it up) to assess its validity (closeness to the truth) and usefulness (clinical applicability);
4 to implement the results of this appraisal in our clinical practice; and
5 to evaluate our performance.

Hence, evidence-based medicine requires you not only to read papers, but also to read the *right* papers at the right time, and then to alter your behaviour (and, what is often more difficult, influence the behaviour of other people) in the light of what you have found. I am concerned that the plethora of how-to-do-it courses in evidence-based medicine so often concentrate on the third of these five steps (critical appraisal) to the exclusion of all the others. Yet if you have asked the wrong question or sought answers from the wrong sources, you might as well not read any papers at all. Equally, all your training in search techniques and critical appraisal will go to waste if you do not put at least as much effort into implementing valid evidence and measuring progress towards your goals as you do into reading the paper.

If I were to be pedantic about the title of this book, these broader aspects of evidence-based medicine should not even get a mention here. But I hope you would have demanded your money back if I had omitted the final section of this chapter (Before you start: formulate the problem), Chapter 2 (Searching the literature) and Chapter 13 (Getting evidence into practice). Chapters 3–12 describe step (3) of the evidence-based medicine process: critical appraisal – that is, what you should do when you actually have the paper in front of you.

Incidentally, if you are computer literate and want to explore the subject of evidence-based medicine on the Internet, you could try the following websites. If you're not, don't worry (and don't worry either when you discover that there are over 200 websites dedicated to evidence-based medicine – they all offer very similar material and you certainly don't need to visit them all).

1 **Oxford Centre for Evidence-Based Medicine** A well-kept website from Oxford, UK containing a wealth of resources and links for EBM. http://cebm.net

2 **Centre for Health Evidence** An excellent Canadian website linking to a wealth of useful resources and also listing ongoing research projects in evidence-based practice. http://cche.net/che/home.asp

3 **Centre for Evidence-Based Nursing** A site for nurses and those interested in nursing topic areas, led by Professor Nicky Cullum. http://www.york.ac.uk/healthsciences/centres/evidence/cebn.htm

4 **NHS Centre for Reviews and Dissemination** The site for downloading the high-quality evidence-based reviews in the National Health Service (NHS) funded 'Effective Health Care' series – a good starting point when looking for evidence on complex questions such as 'what should we do about obesity?' http://www.york.ac.uk/inst/crd

5 **Clinical Evidence** An online version of the excellent 6-monthly handbook of best evidence for clinical decisions such as what's the best current treatment for atrial fibrillation? Produced by the BMJ Publishing Group. http://www.clinicalevidence.com

1.2 Why do people often groan when you mention evidence-based medicine?

Critics of evidence-based medicine might define it as 'the increasingly fashionable tendency of a group of young, confident and highly numerate medical academics to belittle the performance of experienced clinicians using a combination of epidemiological jargon and statistical sleight-of-hand', or 'the argument, usually presented with near-evangelistic zeal, that no health-related action should ever be taken by a doctor, a nurse, a manager of health services, or a politician, unless and until the results of several large and expensive research trials have appeared in print and approved by a committee of experts'.

Others have put their reservations even more strongly: 'evidence-based medicine seems to (replace) original findings with subjectively selected, arbitrarily summarised, laundered, and biased conclusions of indeterminate validity or completeness. It has been carried out by people of unknown ability, experience, and skills using methods whose opacity prevents assessment of the original data'.[3]

The palpable resentment amongst many health professionals towards the evidence-based medicine movement [3–5] is mostly a reaction to the implication that doctors (and nurses, midwives, physiotherapists and other health professionals) were functionally illiterate until they were shown the light, and that the few who weren't illiterate wilfully ignored published medical evidence. Anyone who works face to face with patients knows how often it is necessary to seek new information before making a clinical decision. Doctors have spent time in libraries since libraries were invented. We don't put a patient on a new drug without evidence that it is likely to work. Apart from anything else, such off-licence use of medication is, strictly speaking, illegal. Surely we have all been practising evidence-based medicine for years, except when we were deliberately bluffing (using the 'placebo' effect for good medical reasons), or when we were ill, overstressed or consciously being lazy?

Well, no, we haven't. There have been a number of surveys on the behaviour of doctors, nurses and related professionals. It was estimated in the 1970s in the United States that only around 10–20% of all health technologies then available (i.e. drugs, procedures, operations and so on) were evidence based; this figure improved to 21% in 1990, according to official U.S. statistics.[6] More recently, researchers seem to have stopped looking at technologies that are actually used for particular patient care decisions. Studies of the interventions offered to consecutive series of patients have suggested that 60–90% of clinical decisions, depending on the specialty, are 'evidence based'.[7–11] But as I have argued elsewhere,[12] these studies had methodological limitations. Apart from anything else, they were undertaken in specialised units and looked at the practice of world experts in evidence-based medicine; hence, the figures arrived at can hardly be generalised beyond their immediate setting (see Section 4.2).

Let's take a look at the various approaches that health professionals use to reach their decisions in reality – all of which are examples of what evidence-based medicine *isn't*.

Decision-making by anecdote

When I was a medical student, I occasionally joined the retinue of a distinguished professor as he made his daily ward rounds. On seeing a new patient, he would enquire about the patient's symptoms, turn to the massed ranks of juniors around the bed, and relate the story of a similar patient encountered a few years previously. 'Ah, yes. I remember we gave her such-and-such, and she was fine after that'. He was cynical, often rightly, about new drugs and technologies and his clinical acumen was second to none. Nevertheless, it had taken him 40 years to accumulate his expertise, and the largest medical textbook of all – the collection of cases that were outside his personal experience – was forever closed to him.

Anecdote (storytelling) has an important place in clinical practice.[13] Psychologists have shown that students acquire the skills of medicine, nursing and so on by memorising what was wrong with particular patients, and what happened to them, in the form of stories or 'illness scripts'. Stories about patients are the 'unit of analysis' (i.e. the thing we study) in grand rounds and teaching sessions. Clinicians glean crucial information from patients' illness narratives – most crucially, perhaps, what being ill *means* to the patient.[14] And experienced doctors and nurses rightly take account of the accumulated 'illness scripts' of all their previous patients when managing subsequent patients. But that doesn't mean simply doing the same for patient B as you did for patient A if your treatment worked, and doing precisely the opposite if it didn't!

The dangers of decision-making by anecdote are well illustrated by considering the risk–benefit ratio of drugs and medicines. In my first pregnancy, I developed severe vomiting and was given the anti-sickness drug prochlorperazine (Stemetil). Within minutes, I went into an uncontrollable and very distressing neurological spasm. Two days later I recovered fully from this idiosyncratic reaction, but I have never prescribed the drug since, even though the estimated prevalence of neurological reactions to prochlorperazine is only one in several thousand cases. Conversely, it is tempting to dismiss the possibility of rare but potentially serious adverse effects from familiar drugs – such as thrombosis on the contraceptive pill – when one has never encountered such problems in oneself or one's patients.

We clinicians would not be human if we ignored our personal clinical experiences, but we would be better to base our decisions on the collective experience of thousands of clinicians treating millions of patients, rather than on what we as individuals have seen and felt. Chapter 5 of this book (Statistics for the non-statistician) describes some more objective methods, such as the number needed to treat (NNT), for deciding whether a particular drug (or other intervention) is likely to do a patient significant good or harm.

When the evidence-based medicine movement was still in its infancy, Dave Sackett emphasised that evidence-based practice was no threat to old-fashioned clinical experience or judgement.[1] The question of *how* clinicians can manage to be both 'evidence based' (i.e. systematically informing their decisions by research evidence) and 'narrative based' (i.e. embodying all the richness of their accumulated clinical anecdotes and treating each patient's problem as a unique illness story rather than as a 'case of X') is a difficult one to address philosophically, and is beyond the scope of this book. The interested reader might like to look up two articles I've written on this topic[15,16].

Decision-making by press cutting

For the first 10 years after I qualified, I kept an expanding file of papers that I had ripped out of my medical weeklies before binning the less interesting parts. If an article or editorial seemed to have something new to say, I consciously altered my clinical practice in line with its conclusions. Since one article said that all children with suspected urinary tract infections should be sent for kidney scans to exclude congenital abnormalities I began referring anyone under the age of 16 with urinary symptoms for specialist investigations. The advice was in print, and it was recent, so it must surely replace what had been standard practice – in this case, referring only children below the age of 10 who had two well-documented infections.

This approach to clinical decision-making is still very common. How many doctors do you know who justify their approach to a particular clinical problem by citing the results section of a single published study, even though they could not tell you anything at all about the methods used to obtain these results? Was the trial randomised and controlled (see Section 3.6)? How many patients, of what age, sex and disease severity, were involved (see Section 4.2)? How many withdrew from ('dropped out of') the study, and why (see Section 4.6)? By what criteria were patients judged cured (see Section 6.3)? If the findings of the study appeared to contradict those of other researchers, what attempt was made to validate (confirm) and replicate (repeat) them (see Section 7.3)? Were the statistical tests that allegedly proved the authors' point appropriately chosen and correctly performed (see Chapter 5)? Doctors (and nurses, midwives, medical managers, psychologists, medical students and consumer activists) who like to cite the results of medical research studies have a responsibility to ensure that they first go through a checklist of questions like these (more of which are listed in Appendix 1).

Decision-making by GOBSAT (good old boys sat around a table)

When I wrote the first edition of this book in the mid-1990s, the commonest sort of guideline was what was known as a consensus statement – the fruits of a weekend's hard work by a dozen or so eminent experts who had been shut in a luxury hotel, usually at the expense of a drug company. Such 'GOBSAT guidelines' often fell out of the medical freebies (free medical journals and other 'information sheets' sponsored either directly or indirectly by the pharmaceutical industry) as pocket-sized booklets replete with potted recommendations and at-a-glance management guides. But who says the advice given in a set of guidelines, a punchy editorial, or an amply-referenced overview is correct?

Professor Cynthia Mulrow, one of the founders of the science of systematic review (see Chapter 8), has shown that experts in a particular clinical field are actually *less* likely to provide an objective review of all the available evidence than a non-expert who approaches the literature with unbiased eyes.[17] In extreme cases, an 'expert opinion' may consist simply of the lifelong bad habits and personal press cuttings of an ageing clinician, and a gaggle of such experts would simply multiply the misguided views of any one of them. Table 1.1 gives examples of practices that were at one time widely accepted as good clinical practice (and which would have made it into the GOBSAT guideline of the day), but that have subsequently been discredited by high-quality clinical trials.[18]

Chapter 8 of this book takes you through a checklist for assessing whether a 'systematic review of the evidence' produced to support recommendations for practice or policy making really merits the description, and Chapter 9 discusses the harm that can be done by applying guidelines that are not evidence based. It is a major achievement of the evidence-based medicine movement that almost no guideline these days is produced by GOBSAT!

Decision-making by cost minimisation

The general public is usually horrified when it learns that a treatment has been withheld from a patient for reasons of cost. Managers, politicians and, increasingly, doctors can count on being pilloried by the press when a child with a rare cancer is not sent to a specialist unit in America or a frail old lady is denied preventive therapy for osteoporosis. Yet in the real world, all health care is provided from a limited budget and it is increasingly recognised that clinical decisions must take into account the economic costs of a given intervention. As Chapter 10 argues, clinical decision-making *purely* on the grounds of cost ('cost minimisation' – purchasing the cheapest option with no regard to how effective it is) is usually both senseless and cruel, and we are right to object vocally when this occurs.

Expensive interventions should not, however, be justified simply because they are new, or because they ought to work in theory, or because the only alternative is to do nothing – but because they are very likely to

Table 1.1 Examples of harmful practices once strongly supported by 'expert opinion'

Approximate time period	Clinical practice accepted by experts of the day	Research evidence showing the practice to be harmful	Impact on clinical practice
From 500 BC	Blood letting (for just about any acute illness)	1820*	Blood letting ceased around 1910
1957	Thalidomide for 'morning sickness' in early pregnancy, which led to the birth of over 8000 severely malformed babies worldwide	1960	The teratogenic effects of this drug were so dramatic that thalidomide was rapidly withdrawn when the first case report appeared
From at least 1900	Bed rest for acute low back pain	1986	Many doctors still advise people with back pain to 'rest up'
1960s	Benzodiazepines (e.g. diazepam) for mild anxiety and insomnia, initially marketed as 'non-addictive' but subsequently shown to cause severe dependence and withdrawal symptoms	1975	Benzodiazepine prescribing for these indications fell in the 1990s
1970s	Intravenous lignocaine in acute myocardial infarction, with a view to preventing arrhythmias, subsequently shown to have no overall benefit and in some cases to *cause* fatal arrhythmias	1974	Lignocaine continued to be given routinely until the mid-1980s

*Interestingly, blood letting was probably the first practice for which a randomised controlled trial was suggested. The physician Van Helmont issued this challenge to his colleagues as early as 1662: 'Let us take 200 or 500 poor people that have fevers. Let us cast lots, that one half of them may fall to my share, and the others to yours. I will cure them without blood-letting, but you do as you know – and we shall see how many funerals both of us shall have'.[18] I am grateful to Matthias Egger for drawing my attention to this example.

save life or significantly improve its quality. How, though, can the benefits of a hip replacement in a 75-year-old be meaningfully compared with that of cholesterol-lowering drugs in a middle-aged man or of infertility investigations for a couple in their twenties? Somewhat counter-intuitively, there is no self-evident set of ethical principles or analytical tools that we can use to match limited resources to unlimited demand. As we see in Chapter 10, the much-derided quality adjusted life year (QALY) and similar utility-based units are simply attempts to lend some objectivity to the illogical but unavoidable comparison of apples with oranges in the field of human suffering. In the United Kingdom, the National Institute for Clinical Excellence (see www.nice.org.uk) seeks to develop both evidence-based guidelines and fair allocation of National Health Service resources; its work is discussed further in Chapters 9 and 10.

There is one more reason why some people find the term 'evidence-based medicine' unpalatable. This chapter has argued that evidence-based medicine is about coping with change, not about knowing all the answers before you start. In other words, it is not so much about what you have read in the past, but about how you go about identifying and meeting your ongoing learning needs and applying your knowledge appropriately and consistently in new clinical situations. Doctors who were brought up in the old school style of never admitting ignorance may find it hard to accept that a major element of scientific uncertainty exists in practically every clinical encounter, though in most cases, the clinician fails to identify the uncertainty or to articulate it in terms of an answerable question (see Section 1.3). If you're interested in the research evidence on doctors' (lack of) questioning behaviour, refer to Deborah Swinglehurst[19] for an excellent recent review.

The fact that none of us – not even the cleverest or most experienced – can answer all the questions that arise in the average clinical encounter means that the 'expert' is more fallible than he or she was traditionally cracked up to be. An evidence-based approach to ward rounds may turn the traditional medical hierarchy on its head when the staff nurse or junior doctor produces new evidence that challenges what the consultant taught everyone last week. For some senior clinicians, learning the skills of critical appraisal is the least of their problems in adjusting to an evidence-based teaching style!

1.3 Before you start: formulate the problem

When I ask my medical students to write me an essay about high blood pressure, they often produce long, scholarly and essentially correct statements on what high blood pressure is, what causes it and what the treatment options are. On the day they hand in their essays, most of them know far more about high blood pressure than I do. They are certainly aware that high blood pressure is the single most common cause of stroke, and that detecting and treating everyone's high blood pressure would cut the incidence of stroke by almost half. Most of them are aware that stroke, though devastating when it happens, is a fairly rare event, and that blood pressure tablets have side effects such as tiredness, dizziness, impotence and getting 'caught short' when a long way from the lavatory.

But when I ask my students a practical question, such as 'Mrs Jones has developed light-headedness on these blood pressure tablets and she wants to stop all medication; what would you advise her to do'?, they are foxed. They sympathise with Mrs Jones's predicament, but they cannot distil from their pages of close-written text the one thing that Mrs Jones needs to know. As Richard Smith (paraphrasing T.S. Eliot) asked a few years ago in a *BMJ* editorial, 'Where is the wisdom we have lost in knowledge, and the knowledge we have lost in information'?[20].

Experienced doctors (and many nurses) might think they can answer Mrs Jones's question from their own personal experiences. As I argued in the previous section, few of them would be right. And even if they were right on this occasion, they would still need an overall system for converting the rag-bag of information about a patient (an ill-defined set of symptoms, physical signs, test results and knowledge of what happened to this patient or a similar patient the last time), the particular values and preferences (utilities) of the patient and other things that could be relevant (a hunch, a half-remembered article, the opinion of an older and wiser colleague or a paragraph discovered by chance while flicking through a textbook) into a succinct summary of what the problem is and what specific additional items of information we need to solve this problem.

Sackett and colleagues have recently helped us by dissecting the parts of a good clinical question:[21]

• First, define precisely *whom* the question is about (i.e. ask 'How would I describe a group of patients similar to this one'?).

• Next, define *which* manoeuvre you are considering in this patient or population (e.g. a drug treatment), and, if necessary, a comparison manoeuvre (e.g. placebo or current standard therapy).

• Finally, define the desired (or undesired) *outcome* (e.g. reduced mortality, better quality of life, overall cost savings to the health service and so on).

The second step may not, in fact, concern a drug treatment, surgical operation or other intervention. The 'manoeuvre' could, for example, be the exposure to a putative carcinogen (something that might cause cancer) or the detection of a particular surrogate endpoint in a blood test or other investigation. (A surrogate end point, as Section 6.3 explains, is something that predicts, or is said to predict, the later development or progression of disease. In reality, there are very few tests which reliably act as crystal balls for patients' medical future. The statement 'The doctor looked at the test results and told me I had 6 months to live' usually reflects either poor memory or irresponsible doctoring!). In both these cases, the 'outcome' would be the development of cancer (or some other disease) several years later. In most clinical problems with individual patients, however, the manoeuvre consists of a specific intervention initiated by a health professional.

Thus, in Mrs Jones's case, we might ask, 'In a 68-year-old white woman with essential (i.e. common-or-garden) hypertension (high blood pressure), no coexisting illness, and no significant past medical history, do the benefits of continuing therapy with bendrofluazide (chiefly, reduced risk of stroke) outweigh the inconvenience'? Note that in framing the specific question, we have already established that Mrs Jones has never had a heart attack, stroke, or early warning signs such as transient paralysis or loss of vision. If she had, her risk of subsequent stroke would be much higher and we would, rightly, load the risk–benefit equation to reflect this.

In order to answer the question we have posed, we must determine not just the risk of stroke in untreated hypertension, but also the likely reduction in that risk which we can expect with drug treatment. This is, in fact, a rephrasing of a more general question (do the benefits of treatment in this case outweigh the risks?) which we should have asked before we prescribed bendrofluazide to Mrs Jones in the first place, and which all doctors should, of course, ask themselves every time they reach for their prescription pad.

Remember that Mrs Jones' alternative to staying on this particular drug is not necessarily to take no drugs at all; there may be other drugs with equivalent efficacy but less disabling side effects (as Chapter 6 argues, too many clinical trials of new drugs compare the product with placebo rather than with the best available alternative), or non-medical treatments such as exercise, salt restriction, homeopathy or acupuncture. Not all of these approaches would help Mrs Jones or be acceptable to her, but it would be quite appropriate to seek evidence as to *whether* they might help her.

We will probably find answers to some of these questions in the medical literature, and Chapter 2 describes how to search for relevant papers once you have formulated the problem. But before you start, give one last thought to your patient with high blood pressure. In order to determine her personal priorities (how does she value a 10% reduction in her risk of stroke in 5 years' time compared to the inability to go shopping unaccompanied today?), you will need to approach Mrs Jones, not a blood pressure specialist or the Medline database!

Some writers on evidence-based medicine are enthusiastic about using a decision-tree approach to incorporate the patient's perspective into an evidence-based treatment choice.[22] In practice, this often proves impossible, because (I believe) patients' experiences are complex stories that refuse to be reduced to a tree of yes/no decisions. Perhaps the most powerful criticism of evidence-based medicine is that, if misapplied, it dismisses the patient's own perspective on their illness in favour of an average effect on a population sample or a column of QALYs (see Chapter 10) calculated by a medical statistician. In the past few years, the evidence-based medicine movement has made rapid progress in developing a more practical methodology for incorporating the patient's perspective in clinical decision making,[23,24] the introduction of evidence-based policy[25] and the design and conduct of research trials (see the website of INVOLVE – previously known as Consumers in NHS Research http://www.invo.org.uk). I have attempted to incorporate the patient's perspective into Sackett's five-stage model for evidence-based practice[12]; the resulting eight stages, which I have called a context-sensitive checklist for evidence-based practice, are shown in Appendix 1.

EXERCISE 1

1 Go back to the fourth paragraph in this chapter where examples of clinical questions are given. Decide whether each of these is a properly focused question in terms of

a) the patient or problem;

b) the manoeuvre (intervention, prognostic marker, exposure);

c) the comparison manoeuvre, if appropriate; and

d) the clinical outcome.

2 Now try the following:

a) A 5-year-old child has been on high-dose topical steroids for severe eczema since the age of 20 months. The mother believes that the steroids are stunting the child's growth, and wishes to change to homeopathic treatment. What information does the dermatologist need to decide (a) whether she is right about the topical steroids and (b) whether homeopathic treatment will help this child?

b) A woman who is 9 weeks pregnant calls out her GP because of abdominal pain and bleeding. A previous ultrasound scan showed that the pregnancy was not ectopic. The GP decides that she might be having a miscarriage and tells her to go into hospital for a scan and, possibly, an operation to clear out the womb. The woman refuses. What information do they both need in order to establish whether hospital admission is medically necessary?

c) In the United Kingdom, most parents take their babies at the ages of 6 weeks, 8 months, 18 months and 3 years for developmental checks, where a doctor listens for heart murmurs, feels the abdomen and checks that the testicles are present, and a nurse shakes a rattle and counts how many bricks the infant can build into a tower. Ignoring the social aspects of 'well-baby clinics', what information would you need to decide whether the service is a good use of health resources?

References

1 Sackett DL, Rosenberg WC, Gray JAM. Evidence based medicine: what it is and what it isn't. *BMJ* 1996;**312**:71–2.

2 Sackett D, Haynes B. On the need for evidence-based medicine. *Evid Based Med* 1995;**1**:4–5.

3 Stradling JR, Davies RJO. The unacceptable face of evidence-based medicine. *J Eval Clin Pract* 1997;**3**:99–103.

4 Williams DD, Garner J. The case against 'the evidence': a different perspective on evidence-based medicine. *Br J Psychiatry* 2002;**180**:8–12.

5 Cohen AM, Stavri PZ, Hersh WR. A categorization and analysis of the criticisms of evidence-based medicine. *Int J Med Inform* 2004;**73**:35–43.

6 Dubinsky M, Ferguson JH. Analysis of the National Institutes of Health Medicare Coverage Assessment. *Int J Technol Assess Health Care* 1990;**6**:480–8.

7 Howes N, Chagla L, Thorpe M, McCulloch P. Surgical practice is evidence based. *Br J Surg* 1997;**84**:1220–3.

8 Myles PS, Bain DL, Johnson F, McMahon R. Is anaesthesia evidence-based? A survey of anaesthetic practice. *Br J Anaesth* 1999;**82**:591–5.

9 Geddes J, Game D, Jenkins N, Peterson LA, Pottinger GR, Sackett DL. In: patient psychiatric treatment is evidence-based. *Qual Health Care* 1996;**4**:215–17.

10 Gill P, Dowell AC, Neal RD, Smith N, Heywood P, Wilson AE. Evidence-based general practice: a retrospective study of interventions in one training practice. *BMJ* 1996;**312**:819–21.

11 Ellis J, Mulligan I, Rowe J, Sackett DL, Ellis J, Mulligan I, Rowe J, Sackett DL. Inpatient general medicine is evidence-based. *Lancet* 1995;**346**:407–10.

12 Greenhalgh T. 'Is my practice evidence-based?'. *BMJ* 1996;**313**:957–8.

13 Macnaughton J. Anecdote in clinical practice. In: Greenhalgh T, Hurwitz B, eds. *Narrative based medicine: dialogue and discourse in clinical practice.* London: BMJ Publications, 1998.

14 Greenhalgh T, Hurwitz B. Narrative based medicine: why study narrative? *BMJ* 1999;**318**:48–50.

15 Greenhalgh T. Intuition and evidence – uneasy bedfellows? *Br J Gen Pract* 2002;**52**:395–400.

16 Greenhalgh T. Narrative based medicine: narrative based medicine in an evidence based world. *BMJ* 1999;**318**:323–5.

17 Mulrow C. Rationale for systematic reviews. *BMJ* 1995;**309**:597–9.

18 van Helmont JA. *Oriatrike, or physick refined: the common errors therein refuted and the whole art reformed and rectified.* London: Lodowick-Loyd, 1662.

19 Swinglehurst D. Information needs of primary care. *J Inform Prim Care* 2005 (in press).

20 Smith R. Where is the wisdom...? *BMJ* 1991;**303**:798–9.

21 Sackett DL, Richardson WS, Rosenberg WMC, Haynes RB. *Evidence-based medicine: how to practice and teach EBM*, 2nd edn. London: Churchill-Livingstone, 2000.

22 Llewellyn-Thomas HA. Investigating patients' preferences for different treatment options. *Can J Nurs Res* 1997;**29**:45–64.

23 Boote J, Telford R, Cooper C. Consumer involvement in health research: a review and research agenda. *Health Policy* 2002;**61**:213–36.

24 Entwistle VA, O'Donnell M. Research funding organisations and consumer involvement. *J Health Serv Res Policy* 2003;**8**:129–31.

25 Majone G. *Evidence, argument and persuasion in the policy process.* New Haven, CT: Yale University Press, 1989.

Chapter 2 **Searching the literature**

2.1 Searching for evidence: key principles

Navigating one's way through the jungle that calls itself the medical literature is no easy task. You can apply all the rules for reading a paper correctly but if you're reading the wrong paper you might as well be doing something else entirely. There are already over 20 million medical articles available – though libraries these days rarely store paper copies of them. Every month, thousands of medical journals are published worldwide; the number of different journals which now exist solely to summarise articles from these journals probably exceeds 300. Only 10–15% of the material that published today will subsequently prove to be of lasting scientific value. A number of research studies have shown that most clinicians are unaware of the extent of the clinical literature and of how to go about accessing it.[1]

Dr David Jewell, in the book *Critical reading for primary care*, reminds us that there are three levels of reading:[2]

1 *browsing*, in which we flick through books and journals looking for anything that might interest us;

2 *reading for information*, in which we approach the literature looking for answers to a specific question, usually related to a problem we have met in real life; and

3 *reading for research*, in which we seek to gain a comprehensive view of the existing state of knowledge, ignorance and uncertainty in a defined area.

In practice, most of us get most of our information (and, let's face it, a good deal of pleasure) from browsing. To overapply the rules for critical appraisal that follow in the rest of this book would be to kill the enjoyment of casual reading. Jewell warns us, however, to steer a path between the bland gullibility of believing everything and the strenuous intellectualism of formal critical appraisal.

If you are browsing (reading for the fun of it), you can read what you like, in whatever order you wish. If you are reading for information (focused searching) or research (systematic review), you will waste time and miss many valuable articles if you simply search at random. This is why we need databases and indexes: to organize scattered information and bring together articles on specific subjects that may be published in widely different and even unexpected journals.

General searches of databases and indexes can turn up a wide variety of material, everything from elegantly designed multicentre randomized controlled trials and systematic reviews to single case studies, tutorial reviews, and personal opinions. All of them constitute evidence to some degree – the degree of believability, however, varies enormously.

The term 'level of evidence' occurs frequently and refers to just this: how far can I trust the article? Usually the level of evidence corresponds to the study design and the nature of the article, with systematic reviews of randomized controlled trials and well-designed randomized controlled trials at the pinnacle of the evidence pyramid, followed by observational studies such as cohort studies or case-control studies, then case studies, then authority and bench studies somewhere towards the base. Figure 2.1 shows a simplified 'levels of evidence' table. For a more detailed table showing levels of evidence relative to the different domains of clinical questions – therapy, diagnosis, prognosis, harm – click 'levels of evidence' at http://www.eboncall.org/.

When I wrote the first edition of this book in 1995, I was pretty confident of taking the reader through database searching using my own rather pragmatic tricks of the trade. But in the intervening years, searching has become a very sophisticated science, and the new version of this chapter owes much to

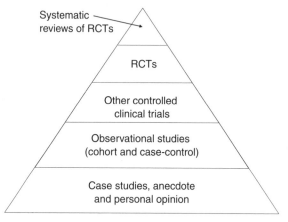

Figure 2.1 A simple hierarchy of evidence for assessing the quality of trial design in therapy studies.

the input of a specialist librarian Jeanette Buckingham from the University of Alberta, Canada. Jeanette has been teaching EBM to medical students, doctors and nurses for many years, and I'm most grateful to her for helping to convey what has become a very specialist knowledge area.

2.2 Medline and other 'raw' databases

Many (but not all) medical articles are indexed in the huge Medline database (Box 2.1). Medline is compiled by the National Library of Medicine (NLM) in the United States and indexes over 5000 journals published in over 70 countries and comprises more than 15 million records. Medline is available online on the World Wide Web, either via the NLM PubMed interface or from commercial vendors who impose their own search engines, or on CD-ROM sets of around 20 CDs. Standard Medline is available from 1966 to the present, 'Old Medline' from 1950 to 1965, and a separate PreMedline database covers new and otherwise unprocessed and unindexed articles.

The Medline database is virtually the same however it is accessed, but the methods of searching it differ depending on the provider's search engine. PubMed is accessible free worldwide on the Internet, http://www.ncbi.nlm.nih.gov/PubMed/. Commercial vendors of Medline either online or CD-ROM include Ovid Technologies (Ovid and WinSPIRS) and Aries Systems Inc (Knowledge Finder).

The best way to learn to use Medline is to book a session with a professional librarian, informaticist or other person experienced with the database. Online tutorials are also readily available. Unless you are a technophobe, you can pick up the basics in less than an hour. Remember that you can search for articles

---

Box 2.1 Examples of 'raw' databases and indexes

'old' Medicine
AMED
CINAHL
Current contents
Embase
Health Star
Medicine
Pre-medicine
PsychInfo

Note also the useful search engine Google Scholar

in two ways:

1 By any word included in the record – including words in the title, abstract, authors' names, and the institution where the research was done. (The abstract is a short summary of what the article is all about, which you will find on the database as well as at the beginning of the printed article.) References can also be traced by numerical identifiers, such as page or volume numbers or by accession numbers or 'universal identifiers'.

2 By a controlled vocabulary or thesaurus of medical titles, known as medical subject heading (MeSH) terms and their accompanying sub-headings. The value of searching by MeSH headings, the indexing terms attached to individual Medline records, is that the same term is used consistently for the same concept, which may have an array of possible synonyms. Because of its organization, in a kind of 'tree', MeSH headings also allow you to search generically – for example, all heart diseases or all non-steroidal anti-inflammatory drugs (NSAIDS) rather than having to list each one.

Entry of articles onto the Medline database is open to human error, both from authors/editors, who write the titles and abstracts, and from indexers who apply MeSH terms and subheadings. Furthermore, a great many important medical and paramedical journals are not covered by Medline at all, particularly journals not published in the United States. Medline lacks comprehensive references in several fields, including psychology, medical sociology, occupational and environmental health, rehabilitation disciplines, and non-clinical pharmacology. If you wish to broaden your search to other electronic databases, ask your local librarian where you can access the other databases listed in Boxes 2.1–2.7.

Here are details of some databases you might wish to explore if your specialist interest is in an appropriate area:

1 *Allied and Complementary Medicine (AMED)* Covers a range of complementary and alternative medicine including homeopathy, chiropractic, acupuncture and so on. Produced by the British Library, available from a number of suppliers including SilverPlatter or Ovid. For more details on AMED, see http://www.silverplatter.com.catalog/amed.htm

2 *CINAHL* The nursing and allied health database covering all aspects of nursing, health education, occupational therapy, social services in health care and other related disciplines from 1983. The CD-ROM version is updated monthly. www.cinahl.com

3 *Current Contents Search* Indexes journal tables of content on or before their publication date. It is useful when checking for the very latest output on a subject. Updated weekly. From 1990. Available from Ovid http://ovid.gwdg.de/ovidweb/fldguide/cc.htm#geni or from Thomson ISI http://www.isinet.com/.

4 *Embase* The database of Excerpta Medica which focuses on drugs and pharmacology, clinical medicine and other biomedical specialties. It is more up-to-date than Medline, with more detailed indexing and better European coverage. Available via a number of database suppliers including Ovid (see reference list).

5 *HealthSTAR* (1975 to 2002) Covers an international range of journals, books, book chapters and technical reports in the areas of health services and hospital administration and health technology assessment. Topics include health economics; financial and personnel administration in the health sector; quality assurance and assessment; materials management in health institutions; health policy; health services planning; evaluation of patient outcomes; effectiveness of procedures, programmes, products and processes. The coverage is international, but U.S. literature is prevalent. Sadly, this database is no longer being updated.

6 *PsycInfo* Produced by the American Psychological Association as the computer-searchable version of Psychological Abstracts. It covers psychology, psychiatry and related subjects; journals are included from 1806 and books from 1987 (English language only). Available through several database vendors, including Ovid (see reference list).

7 *SCOPUS* Searches titles, abstracts and keywords of 14,000 science, technology and medical journals, as well as patents and the Web. Citation links are provided for the articles, and links are also provided to the full text document. Very broad international coverage.

As well as databases, note the increasing value of search engines, especially the following:

1 *Google (and particularly Google Scholar)* Simplistic as it sounds, Google has evolved into an effective search tool for full text peer reviewed journals that are online, not just open access journals or other websites. Ranking the relevance of the site and inclusion of search filters like 'Randomized controlled trial' or 'systematic review' in the search statement will help retrieve good evidence from this resource. Electronic textbook chapters and resources such as *e-medicine* will also emerge from a Google search.

To illustrate how Medline (and comparable databases) work, I have worked through some common problems in searching in Section 2.10. The scenarios were originally drawn up using Ovid software (see http://www.ovid.com), but I have included notes on WinSPIRS and PubMed. All these systems are designed to be used with what is referred to as Boolean logic – that is, linking particular words (such as 'hypertension', 'therapy' and so on) with operators such as AND, OR and NOT that indicate the relationship of these concepts to each other. Knowledge Finder (see http://www.kfinder.com/newweb/) is a different Medline search software that is marketed as a 'fuzzy logic' system –

Box 2.2 Search filters associated with databases

Clinical queries (PubMed)

TRIP

---

in other words, it is designed to cope with complete questions such as 'what is the best therapy for hypertension'?, and is said to be more suited to the user with little or no training. The practical exercises included at the end of the chapter are all equally possible with all types of Medline software.

2.3 Databases with search filters

In order to extract higher levels of evidence (especially RCTs and other high-quality clinical research trials) from the dross resulting from a straight subject search on Medline or other databases, you generally need to combine your search statement with a 'filter' (Box 2.2). Filters may be simple or complex, but basically they derive from words describing study designs (e.g. 'randomized controlled trial' or 'double blind') or terms associated with good comparative studies (e.g. 'sensitivity', 'specificity', 'likelihood', 'diagnostic accuracy'). Some databases have filters built in for you; with others, you have to type in the instructions manually.

The simplest way to apply a search filter is to search 'Clinical Queries' in PubMed. Filters based on those developed for PubMed Clinical Queries are also available on Ovid Medline as 'limit' keys. In Clinical Queries, select the domain of the question (therapy, diagnosis, prognosis, harm – see Chapter 3 if you're not sure what these terms mean), whether you wish your search to be sensitive (meaning broad) or specific (meaning narrow and highly focused), and enter your very basic search terms. The search engine then adds a filter appropriate to the domain, and the result is – hopefully – a useful list of relevant published clinical research.

It's usually not too difficult to work out by trial and error whether you need a 'specific' or a 'sensitive' search filter. If you're searching on a topic where hardly any papers have been published, you usually want to make your search as broad (sensitive) as possible so as to capture everything, even if this means looking through lots of irrelevant articles. But in mainstream clinical topics, try a sensitive search first and broaden it only if you don't find what you're looking for.

A TRIP search directs you quickly to the best evidence among journal articles, plus practice guidelines, e-textbooks, patient information and allows you to limit your search to the 'Big 4': *BMJ, Lancet, Journal of the American Medical Association* (*JAMA*), and *New England Journal of Medicine.* Access it

Box 2.3 Databases of pre-appraised articles

Cochrane Controlled Clinical Trials Register
Evidence-based digests – for example
- Evidence-Based Cardiology
- Evidence-Based Eye Care
- Evidence-Based Medicine
- Evidence-Based Mental Health
- Evidence-Based Nursing

Health Technology Assessment (HTA) Database
NHS Economic Evaluation Database

at http://www.tripdatabase.com/. My own postgraduate students prefer TRIP to any other database, so it's worth checking out.

2.4 Databases of pre-appraised articles

Another method of extracting clinical research from the great mass of published articles is to use 'pre-appraised' resources. These are generally fairly small databases listing clinical research papers that someone has already selected as being worthy of notice. Two good and very different examples are the Cochrane Central Registry of Controlled Trials (part of the Cochrane Library) and the various digests of clinical articles now available by subject (see Box 2.3).

When I wrote the first edition of this book, the Cochrane Library was a small and exploratory project, but it has now replaced Medline as the clinical researcher's first port of call when looking for quality articles and summaries of clinical research. The Cochrane Library now boasts nearly 4,000 peer-reviewed Cochrane systematic reviews, over 5,000 systematic reviews listed in the Database of Abstracts of Reviews of Effects (DARE), and almost a half-million selected published clinical trials in their Central Registry of Controlled Trials. The story behind the Cochrane project is worth telling.

In 1972, epidemiologist Archie Cochrane called for the establishment of a central international register of clinical trials. (It was Cochrane who, as a rebellious young medical student, marched through the streets of London in 1938 bearing a placard which stated, 'All effective treatments should be free'. His book *Effectiveness and efficiency* caused little reaction at the time but captures the essence of today's evidence-based medicine movement.[3])

Though he never lived to see the eponym, Archie Cochrane's vision of a 100% accurate medical database, the Cochrane Library, is now a reality.

It includes
- *Cochrane Registry of Controlled Trials.*
- *Cochrane Review Methodology Database* – containing articles on the science of research synthesis.
- *Health Technology Assessment Database* – reports of systematic reviews funded by the UK Health Technology Assessment Programme (which can generally be replied upon to produce very high quality reviews)
- *NHS Economic Evaluation Database* – a database of economic evaluations of high-quality clinical trials.

In addition, the Cochrane Library includes two databases of synthesised evidence (Cochrane Database of Systematic Reviews and Database of Abstracts of Reviews of Effectiveness) discussed in Section 2.5.

Published articles are entered onto the Cochrane databases by members of the Cochrane Collaboration, an international network of (mostly) medically qualified volunteers.[4] Using strict methodological criteria, the reviewers classify each article according to publication type (randomised trial, other controlled clinical trial, epidemiological survey and so on), and prepare structured abstracts in house style. The Collaboration has already identified well over 100,000 trials that had not been appropriately tagged in Medline or that were published before Medline had publication types to help identify randomized controlled trials.

In 1997 some of the founder members of the Cochrane Collaboration published a compilation of articles reflecting on Cochrane's original vision and the projects that have emerged from it. Despite its uninspiring title, 'Non-random reflections on health services research is a fascinating account of one of medicine's most important collaborative initiatives in the twentieth century.[5] Finally, if you are interesting in becoming involved with Cochrane Collaboration projects, contact the Cochrane groups and entities via http://www.cochrane.org/index0.htm/

The Cochrane Library also contains useful information about the Cochrane Collaboration and its subject-based review groups and methods – including how to join one and start doing your own systematic review! Since all these databases can be searched together, the Cochrane Library is often a good place to begin a comprehensive search on a clinical topic.

Now for evidence-based digests. You may be familiar with the paper versions of journals like *ACP Journal Club, Evidence-Based Medicine, Evidence-Based Mental Health* and so on. These digests are compilations of articles by interested EBM practitioners, often with a commentary by a subject expert. An editorial board for these digests selects and commisssions critical appraisals of studies published in core journals in the field. This is useful in and of itself, but even better: these journals can be searched like databases and can provide excellent filtered sources for high-level evidence.

Box 2.4 Databases of synthesised evidence

American College of Physicians PIER
Clinical Evidence
Cochrane Database of Systematic Reviews (CDSR)
Database of Abstracts of Reviews of Effectiveness (DARE)
Evidence-Based On Call (EBOC)

2.5 Databases of synthesised evidence

As mentioned above briefly, the Cochrane Library contains two databases of reviews (Box 2.4):

1 *Cochrane Database of Systematic Reviews* (CDSR) This is the gold standard database for synthesised evidence. A particular strength of the CDSR is that authors of systematic reviews undertake to update their own contributions periodically (though this doesn't always happen in practice).

2 *Database of Abstracts of Reviews of Effectiveness* (DARE) – a database and critical appraisal of non-Cochrane systematic reviews published in journals.

If you're a jobbing clinician looking for a quick answer to a clinical question, you might find the idea of these Cochrane review databases somewhat daunting – though you shouldn't dismiss this source since you can often answer specific queries quickly by searching Cochrane abstracts.

Note also these guideline databases:

1 *National Guideline Clearinghouse* This is a comprehensive, U.S.-based database of evidence-based clinical practice guidelines, not only those published in the United States. It permits tabular comparison of guidelines on similar topics, including comparison of levels of evidence for recommendations. Find it on http://www.guideline.gov/

2 *National Institute for Health and Clinical Excellence* (NICE) This government-funded U.K. body is developing a set of nationally approved evidence-based guidelines to support U.K. national health policy. Some are developed in-house by NICE committees, but others are produced externally and appraised and endorsed by NICE. See www.nice.org.uk

Another way of finding high-quality synthesised evidence to support practice is to use sources that not only synthesize the best available evidence but also present it in readily usable formats. Here are some:

1 *Clinical Evidence* In the United Kingdom, this succinct synthesis of best evidence on mainstream clinical areas is sent free in book format to every doctor in the National Health Service every 6 months. It is also

available online on http://www.clinicalevidence.com/ceweb/conditions/index.jsp
2 *PIER* An equivalent database from the American College of Physicians.
3 *Evidence-Based On-Call (EBOC)* – designed for junior doctors on call, this database contains evidence-based summaries of the management of around 40 acute conditions. http://www.eboncall.org/
4 *Book sources* A wealth of evidence-based textbooks and handbooks, most of them online, now exist. Ask your local librarian for the current market leader.
5 *PDAs* A developing subset of synthesized information for evidence-based practice consists of various resources developed for use in hand-held 'Personal Digital Assistants'. The future of evidence-based practice will see more emphasis on synthesized 'point-of-care' resources.

2.6 Databases of ongoing research

If you're doing a systematic review (see Chapter 8) or even what we call a 'quasi-systematic' review (i.e. a review that tries hard to include all relevant sources but which, perhaps because of time constraints, falls short of comprehensive coverage), you might like to flag ongoing research that is due to be reported in the next few months or years (Box 2.5). For this, you'd need something like the UK National Research Register – a register of all RCTs being undertaken, which should now be logged from inception to completion. See http://www.update-software.com/National/

The *BMJ* has recently said that it will not publish RCTs that have not been entered onto the National Research Register. Scientists both within and outside the UK are also strangly encouraged to assign a unique identification number to their study before it commences, to allow it be readily tracked as work unfolds. This can be done at the Current Controlled Trials web site http://www.controlled-trials.com/

2.7 Citation searching

Checking out the references of a particularly good paper or chapter is a time-honoured way of finding highly relevant information. What about taking this concept and turning it forwards in time: who has cited this article in their

---

Box 2.5 Databases of ongoing research

UK National Research Register
Current Controlled Trials

lists of references? This has been done since the 1960s by the Institute for Scientific Information, starting with Science Citation Index, followed by the Social Science Citation Index and Arts and Humanities Citation Index, and has come into its own with the electronic version of these indexes, Web of Science. More recently, Ovid Medline has introduced citation tracking, and Scopus, a relatively new index that searches journals, patents and the Web simultaneously, includes citation tracking as one of its features (Box 2.6).

Citation databases work by indexing the references cited in articles as well as the usual author, title, abstract and citation of the articles themselves. Web of Science is available at http://wos.mimas.ac.uk/

What kind of information do you get from citation tracking?

1 You can follow studies forward in time, to see if there are new studies on a similar or related topic.
2 You can determine how important a study was based on the number of times it has been cited.
3 You can track post-publication peer review, in the form of letters to the editor and commentary, whether in the same journal a paper was published in or in other journals.
4 You can find the address of an author if you want to contact him or her.

An outgrowth of citation searching has been 'related record' searching, available on PubMed Medline and on Web of Science – finding articles that share articles cited as well as an array of keywords. Both are surprisingly effective ways of finding needles in haystacks, and both are very simple indeed.

2.8 Human contact sources

When I did a systematic review of a highly complex area of evidence recently, a total of 495 papers (and books) were listed in the final report. Just out of curiosity, I had collected details on where we had found each of these references – database searching, hand searching, pursuing references of papers we already had or asking our friends. Rather to my surprise, 23% of sources were known to me or to my co-authors, or had been recommended by our academic

---

Box 2.6 Citation searching

Web of Science
   Science Citation Index
   Social Science Citation Index
   Arts and Humanities Citation Index
OVID Medline citation track function
PubMed 'related articles' function

Box 2.7 Human contact sources
CHAIN
Academic mailing lists (see www.jiscmail.ac.uk) – for example
Evidence-based health
Public health

colleagues when we approached them either in person or by email. In other words, we got nearly a quarter of our key papers from asking around![6]

While I would certainly not recommend 'asking around' as a definitive or sole search strategy, I do think the human element deserves more emphasis (Box 2.7). The point is, experts in the field might know of articles in obscure sources – especially what is known as 'grey literature' – that is, papers of potentially high quality that are either unpublished or published only as internal reports (a good example being PhD theses). Apart from your friends and family, good sources of human input for your review might be conference delegates lists, academic email lists or (in the United Kingdom and Canada) the CHAIN (Contact, Help, Advice, Information and Networking) initiative which comprises a website, contact list and centrally facilitated email service. My own team evaluated what people got out of their membership of CHAIN – one prominent theme in our findings was finding 'grey literature' sources of evidence and getting help with implementing EBM in practice.[7] You can join CHAIN for free on http://chain.ulcc.ac.uk/chain/

2.9 Worked examples of search problems

Problem 1: You are trying to find a particular paper which you know exists
Solution: Search the database by field suffix (title, author, journal, institution, etc.) or by textwords.
This shouldn't take long. You do not need to do a comprehensive subject search. Get into the part of the database which covers the approximate year of the paper's publication (usually the past 5 years) – or, if you can't do that easily, just search the entire database back to 1966: the most recent articles are usually displayed at the beginning of your results set.

If you are using the free version of Medline (PubMed) and if you know the title of the paper, simply type it in. If you're using Ovid, you can do this too – for best results, use the title search key *or* enter the title in parentheses followed by the .ti. field label. If you know the journal in which the paper was published, you can also use the .jn. field label. Box 2.8 shows some useful Ovid field labels, most of which are self-explanatory. But note the '.ui.' suffix

---

Box 2.8 Useful search field labels (Ovid Medline)

Syntax	Meaning	Example
.ab.	Word in abstract	epilepsy.ab.
.au.	Author	smith-r.au.
.jn.	Journal	lancet.jn.
.me.	Single word, wherever it may appear as a MeSH term	ulcer.me.
.sh.	Exact MeSH heading	lung neoplasms.sh.
.ti.	Word in title	epilepsy.ti.
.tw.	Word in title or abstract	epilepsy.tw.
.ui.	Unique identifier	91574637.ui.
.yr.	Year of publication	87.yr.

---

which denotes the unique number used to identify a particular Medline entry. If you find an article that you might wish to call up again, it's often quicker to write down the unique identifier rather than the author, title, journal and so on.

To illustrate the use of field labels, let's say you are trying to find a paper called 'A survey of cervical cancer screening in people with learning disability', which you remember seeing in the *BMJ* a few years ago. Make sure you have NOT ticked the Box 2. 'Map term to subject heading', and then type the following into the computer:

> **1 cervical cancer.ti.**

This gives you approximately 6000 possible articles in set 1. Now type

> **2 survey.ti.**

This gives you approximately 47,000 possible articles in set 2. Now type

> **3 learning disability.ti.**

This gives you approximately 525 possible articles in set 3. Now type

> **4 BMJ.jn.**

This gives you almost 40,000 articles in set 4 – that is, all articles from the *BMJ* listed in this part of the Medline database for the years you selected. Now combine these sets, using the combine function on the search page or by typing

5   1 and 2 and 3 and 4

This gives you anything with 'cervical cancer' and 'survey' and 'learning disability' in the title AND which was published in the *BMJ*.[8] You could have also done all the above in one step:

> **(cervical cancer AND survey AND learning disability).ti. AND BMJ.jn.**

This step illustrates the use of the Boolean operator AND, which will give you articles common to both sets. Using the operator OR will retrieve everything in both sets.

You should not generally use abbreviations for journal titles in Ovid, but other software packages may use standard abbreviations. Note, however, that some journals have their abbreviated title as their full title – such as *BMJ* after 1988, or *JAMA* (*Journal of the American Medical Association*). If you are not certain of the full title of the journal, use the field label .jw., meaning 'journal word' to search; this is more useful for specific terms, like 'brain surgery' or 'learning disabilities', than it is for general words like 'medical'. Another important point is that searching for title words will only uncover the *exact* word – for example, this search would have missed an article whose title was about learning *disabilities* rather than disability. To address this problem, you need to use a truncation symbol (see below).

Often, you don't know the title of a paper but you know who wrote it. Alternatively, you may have been impressed with an article you have read (or lecture you heard) by a particular author and you want to see what else they have published. Let's try finding Professor Michael Marmot's publications over the past 5 years. Medline never provides authors' given names, only their initials. The syntax is as follows: Type **marmot m.au.** in the search box

This gives you all the articles in this database in which M. Marmot is an author or co-author – approximately 50 papers. If using WinSPIRS, type 'Marmot M'; and if using PubMed, type 'Marmot M' without the field label; you will end up with an identical list on all the packages. Realise that some may be written by Mary Marmot or Montague Marmot – this is a hazard of author searches on Medline. Also, like many authors, Michael is not the only M Marmot in the medical literature, and – another problem – he has a middle initial which he uses inconsistently in his publications. Unless you already know his middle initial, you must use a *truncation symbol* to find it out. On Ovid, this is $; on WinSPIRS and PubMed it is *. Type **marmot-m$.au.**

This gives you about 60 articles which include the previous 35 you found under M Marmot, plus articles by MA Marmot, MD Marmot and another 25 articles by – we've found him – MG Marmot! You can use the truncation symbol to search a stem in a textword search - for example, the syntax electric$.tw. (in Ovid) will uncover articles with 'electric', 'electricity', 'electrical' and so on in the title or abstract.

You could have used the following single-line search statement:

(marmot m or marmot mg).au.

Or you could use the Author browse function on the Ovid search page and check off Marmot M and Marmot MG.

This gives a total of around 60 articles which you now need to browse by hand to exclude any M Marmots other than Professor Michael! Or if you know the author's institution, you could search by institution field. This will give you all the papers which were produced in a particular research institution. For example, search

(withington hospital and manchester).in.

to find all the papers where 'Withington Hospital, Manchester' appears in the 'institution' field (either as the main address where the research was done or as that of one of the co-authors).

If you can't remember the title of the article you want but you know some exact key phrases from the abstract, it might be quicker to search under textwords than MeSH terms (which are explained in the next section). The field labels you need are .ti. (title), .ab. (abstract) and .tw. (textword = either title or abstract).

Medline allows you to 'limit' searches to commonly used fields, subsets and subjects. Publication type is an important limit, as are language, gender, human age groups and journal subsets (like Core Clinical Journals). The search page on Ovid has a 'limit' icon, and PubMed has a 'limit' tab.

EXERCISE 1

1 Try to track down the following articles using as few commands as possible:

a) A systematic review by Craig and colleagues on the measurement of children's temperature in the axilla compared with the rectum published in a major English language journal in about 2000. (Don't forget that the Ovid system needs an initial for the author's name and uses the syntax 'smith r.au.' or 'smith .$.au.')

b) A paper by Professor Marsh's team from Oxford on the effect of pheno-barbital on the frequency of fits. (Note that you do not need the full address of the institution to search under this field.)

c) A paper describing death rates from different causes in participants in the HOPE (Heart Outcomes Prevention Evaluation) study, by Salim Yusuf and colleagues, published in either the *New England Journal of Medicine* or the *Journal of the American Medical Association* (note that Ovid Medline records the former under its full name and the latter as *JAMA*).

d) Two articles published in 1995 in the *American Journal of Medical Genetics* on the inheritance of schizophrenia in Israeli subjects. See if you can find them in a single command using field labels.

2 Trace the series of ongoing articles published in the *Journal of the American Medical Association* from 1992 to date, entitled "Users' Guides to the Medical Literature". Once you've found them, copy them and keep them. Much of the rest of this book is based on these Users' Guides.

3 How many articles can you find by Professor David Sackett, who, like Professor Marmot, uses his middle initial inconsistently?

4 Find out how many articles were published by Fiona Godlee in the *British Medical Journal* in 2005. Remember that to restrict your search to a particular year in Ovid Medline, use the 'limit set' button at the top of the screen and then select 'publication year', or, alternatively, use the field label '.yr.' (e.g. 05.yr.).

Problem 2: You want to answer a very specific clinical question
Solution: Construct a focused (specific) search by combining two or more broad (sensitive) searches.

I was once asked by the mother of a young girl with anorexia nervosa (whose periods had ceased) to prescribe the oral contraceptive pill so as to stop her bones thinning. This seemed like a reasonable request, though there were ethical problems to consider. But is there any evidence that going on the Pill in these circumstances really prevents long-term bone loss? I decided to explore the subject using Medline. To answer this question, you need to search very broadly under 'anorexia nervosa', 'osteoporosis' and 'oral contraceptives'. Making sure that the 'Map text to subject heading' is ticked, type in the search box.

anorexia nervosa

The Ovid system will automatically try to match your request to one of its standard medical subject headings (abbreviated 'MeSH' and colloquially known as 'mesh terms'). Wait a few seconds, and you should see two options on the screen. The first is 'anorexia nervosa' as a MeSH term, and you are offered two additional choices: 'Explode' and 'Focus'. Ignore the 'explode' Box 2 for now (explained later), and consider the 'focus' box. Do you only want articles that are actually *about* anorexia nervosa, or do you want any article that mentions anorexia nervosa in passing? Let's say we do want to restrict to focus. Next, the screen offers us a choice of subheadings, but we'll ignore these for the moment. Select 'Include all subheadings'. You should have about 1200 articles in this set.

If you don't tick the 'map text to subject heading' box, Ovid will default to a textword search for the term 'anorexia nervosa' in the title or abstract. Incidentally, even if you do tick the 'map' box, it will also offer to do a title and abstract search - that is, find you articles with (say) the words 'anorexia nervosa' in the title or abstract even if the article has not been indexed under this MeSH heading. But in general, if your set is already large, you should avoid textword searches and just use the MeSH headings.

If you do choose to include textword searches, the resulting syntax you see on the search screen is

anorexia nervosa.mp. [title, abstract, registry number word, or MeSH]

Similarly, to get articles on osteoporosis (which is also a MeSH term), type 'osteoporosis/' into the search box:

osteoporosis/

You should get about 20,000 articles. Note that in Ovid, if you know that the subject you want is an official MeSH term, you can cut short the mapping process by typing a slash (/) after the word. This can not only save considerable time, but it can also bypass important and useful features of the Medline system. Note also that we have not used an asterisk here because osteoporosis may not be the focus of the article we are looking for.

Finally, put in the term 'oral contraceptives' (without an asterisk and without a slash) to see what the MeSH term here is. The MeSH term is 'contraceptives, oral' (if you had known this you could have used the syntax **contraceptives,oral/** – but don't do this for a reason I'm about to explain).

oral contraceptives

Ovid maps your request to 'contraceptives,oral' and asks you if you want to restrict your set to focus (probably not) and if you want to explode the term. The MeSH terms are like the branches of a tree, with, for example, 'asthma' subdividing into 'asthma in children', 'occupational asthma' and so on. Medline indexers are instructed to index items using the most specific MeSH terms they can. If you just ask for articles on 'asthma', you will miss all the terminal divisions of the branch unless you 'explode' the term. (Note, however, that you can only explode a term *down* the MeSH tree, not upwards).

If you do not tick the explode Box 2 for 'contraceptives,oral', your set will probably only contain around 700 articles, whereas the exploded term contains about 5000! Explode is particularly important when searching for information about drugs or general classes of diseases, such as heart diseases or kidney diseases. A quick route to explode a topic when you know the MeSH term is

exp contraceptives, oral/

If you combine these three sets, either by using their set numbers (e.g. '1 and 2 and 3' in Ovid or '#1 and #2 and #3' in PubMEd) or the combine icon on the search page, you will have searched over 60,000 articles and obtained a very small set of three or four references, including some original research papers and a useful review article.

EXERCISE 2

Try to find a set of fewer than five articles relating to any of the following questions or clinical problems:

1 Is the high prevalence of coronary heart disease in certain ethnic Asian groups attributable to differences in insulin levels?

2 The hypothesis linking vitamin C with cure of the common cold is, apparently, something to do with its role as an antioxidant. Is there any (clinical or theoretical) evidence to support this hypothesis?

3 How should thyrotoxicosis be managed in pregnancy?

4 Make sure you practice finding the MeSH term for each subject, making judicious use of the asterisk to restrict to focus (but only when the set is large), and using the slash to denote what you know is a MeSH term

---

Problem 3: You want to get general information quickly about a well-defined topic

Solution: Use subheadings and/or the 'limit set' options.

This is one of the commonest reasons why we approach Medline in real life. We don't have a particular paper in mind, or a very specific question to ask, and we aren't aiming for an exhaustive overview of the literature. We just want to know, say, what's the latest expert advice on drug treatment for asthma, or whether anything new has been written on malaria vaccines.

Box 2.9 Useful subheadings (Ovid Medline)

Syntax	meaning	Example
/ae	Adverse effects	**thalidomide/ae**
/ci	Chemically induced	**headache/ci**
/co	complications	**measles/co**
/ct	Contraindications (of drug)	**propranolol/ct**
/di	Diagnosis	**glioma/di**
/dt	Drug therapy	**depression/dt**
/ed	Education	**asthma/ed**
/ep	Epidemiology	**poliomyelitis/ep**
/et	Etiology (aetiology)	**asthma/et**
/hi	History	**mastectomy/hi**
/nu	Nursing	**cerebral palsy/nu**
/og	Organisation/administration	**health service/og**
/pc	Prevention and control	**influenza/pc**
/px	Psychology	**diabetes/px**
/rh	Rehabilitation	**hip fractures/rh**
/su	Surgery	**hip fractures/su**
/th	Therapy	**hypertension/th**
/tu	Therapeutic use (of drug)	**aspirin/tu**

One method to accomplish this is to search using MeSH terms and then, if we unearth a large number of articles *but not otherwise*, to use index subheadings. Subheadings are the fine-tuning of the Medline indexing system, and classify articles on a particular MeSH topic into aetiology, prevention, therapy and so on. The most useful ones are listed in Box 2.9 (you don't have to memorise these since the Ovid MeSH search process automatically offers you subheadings to tick, but you can truncate the mapping process and therefore save time if you do happen to know the subheading you need). I tend not to use subheadings myself, since my librarian colleagues tell me that an estimated 50% of articles in Medline are inadequately or incorrectly classified by subheading An alternative approach is to restrict the set by study design using a search filter, as described in Section 2.3.

Note that the subheading /th in Box 2.9 refers to the non-pharmacological therapy of a disease, whereas /dt is used for drug therapy. The subheading /tu is used exclusively for drugs and means 'therapeutic use of'. The subheading /px is used with non-psychiatric diseases as in this example – diabetes/px = psychosocial aspects of diabetes.

Not all subheadings are used in the indexing system for every topic, but rather are specific to the nature of the topic (e.g. is it a disease, or a body part, or a drug?). To find the subheadings for a MeSH term such as asthma, type

1 sh asthma

This command will tell you which subheadings are used in the indexing system for this MeSH term. It gives you a number of options, including diagnosis, economics, ethnology and so on. Looking for an article about drug therapy for asthma, you would choose /dt (drug therapy). You could have typed the single search statement:

2 *asthma/dt

where the asterisk denotes a major focus of the article, the slash denotes a MeSH term and dt means drug therapy. This will give you around 14,000 articles to choose from.

You now need to *limit the set*, so start with the frequently used options for limiting a set which are listed as tick boxes below the table on your screen ('human', 'reviews' and so on. Limit by years of publication is fine, but not really necessary, since the most recent references are displayed first. Be careful of some of these buttons: on Ovid Medline, for example, 'full text' on the limit panel means articles supplied fulltext via Ovid, which may constitute only a fraction of the full text articles available to you. 'Latest update' is useful only if you have done exactly the same search a week previously – otherwise it may miss important references.

Now select the 'limit set' button at the top of the screen., This leads you to additional options, including age groups, publication types and journal or subject subsets, such as nursing or bioethics. These limits can focus your search more precisely and can cut down the set to a number that you can browse through comfortably. It actually doesn't take long to browse through 50 or so articles on the screen – depending on your tolerance, more than 50 can waste your time and/or burn out your critical faculties. It is often better to browse than to rely on the software to give you the best of the bunch. In other words, don't overapply the 'limit set' commands you find in Box 2.10.

Instead of using the 'limit set' function key, you can use direct single-line commands such as

limit 5 to review
limit 5 to human

Box 2.10 Useful 'limit set' options

Core clinical journals	Review articles	English language
Nursing journals	Editorials	Male/female
Dental journals	Abstracts	Human
Publication year		

EXERCISE 3

Try to find a single paper (by browsing a larger set) to give you a quick answer to the following questions:

1 Is hormone replacement therapy ever indicated in women who have had breast cancer in the past?
2 The North American medical literature often mentions Health Maintenance Organizations. What are these?
3 Imagine that you are a medical journalist who has been asked to write an article on screening for prostate cancer. You want two fairly short review articles, from the mainstream medical literature, to use as your sources.
4 Does watching violence on television lead to violent behaviour in children?

Problem 4: Your search gives you lots of irrelevant articles
Solution: Refine your search as you go along in the light of interim results.
Often, a search uncovers dozens of articles that are irrelevant to your question. The Boolean operator NOT can help here. I once undertook a search to identify articles on surrogate endpoints in clinical pharmacology research. I searched Medline not only by MeSH terms but I also wanted to search by textwords to pick up articles that the MeSH indexing system had missed (see Section 2.7). Unfortunately, my search revealed hundreds of articles I didn't want – all on surrogate motherhood. (Surrogate endpoints are explained in Section 6.3 – they are nothing to do with surrogate motherhood!) The syntax to exclude the unwanted articles is as follows:

1 (surrogate NOT mother$).tw.

Deciding to use the 'not' operator is a good example of how you can (and should) refine your search as you go along – much easier than producing the perfect search off the top of your head. Another way of getting rid of irrelevant articles is to narrow your textword search to adjacent words. For example, the term 'home help' includes two very common words linked in a specific context. Link them as follows:

2 home adj help.tw.

where adj means 'adjacent'. Similarly, 'community adj care', 'Macmillan adj nurse'. You can even specify the number of words gap between two linked words, as in

3 community adj2 care.tw.

which would find 'community mental health care' as well as 'community child care' and 'community care'.

EXERCISE 4

1 Find articles about occupational asthma caused by sugar.
2 The drug chloroquine is most commonly used for the treatment of falciparum malaria. Find out what other uses it has. (Hint: use the subheading /tu, which means 'therapeutic use', and remember that malaria is often referred to by its Latin name 'plasmodium falciparum'. You should, of course, limit a large search to review articles if you are reading for quick information rather than secondary research.)

Problem 5: Your search gives you no articles at all, or not as many as you expected
Solution: First, don't overuse subheadings or the 'limit set' options. Second, search under textwords as well as MeSH terms. Third, learn about the 'explode' command, and use it routinely.
If your carefully constructed search bears little or no fruit, it is possible that there are no relevant articles in the database. More likely, you have missed them. Many important articles are missed not because we constructed a flawed search strategy but because we relied too heavily on a flawed indexing system. I've already talked about the overuse of subheadings (see Section 2.5). MeSH terms may also be wrongly assigned, or not assigned at all. Discrepancies arise in particular when the obvious subjects aren't in the abstract. For this reason, you should adopt a 'belt and braces' approach and search under textwords as well as by MeSH. After all, it's difficult to write an article on the psychology of diabetes without mentioning the words 'diabetes', 'diabetic', 'psychology' or 'psychological', so the truncation stems 'diabet$.tw.' and 'psychol$.tw.' would supplement a search under the MeSH term 'diabetes mellitus' and the subheading /px (psychology).

For example, if you wanted to answer the question 'what is the role of aspirin in the prevention and treatment of myocardial infarction', you could type the single-line statement:

1 (myocardial infarction/pc or myocardial infarction/dt) and aspirin/tu

which would give you all articles listed in this part of the Medline database which cover the therapeutic use of aspirin and the prevention or treatment of myocardial infarction – 1260 or so articles, but no immediate answer to your question. You might be better off dropping the subheadings and limiting the set as follows:

1 myocardial infarction/ and aspirin/
2 limit 1 to Core Clinical journals
3 limit 2 to review articles

a strategy which would give you around 99 general review articles, including at least one very useful one which your first search (by subheadings) missed. Note, however, that it would exclude *systematic* reviews, which are (somewhat bizarrely) indexed as 'meta-analyses' in Medline. If you're searching for research purposes (see Section 2.1), you should use the 'meta-analysis' limit key, but if a brief overview of the subject is what you're looking for, 'review articles' will probably suffice.

Now, let's add an extra string to this strategy:

4 (myocardial infarct$ and aspirin).mp
5 1 or 4
6 limit 5 to Core Clinical journals
7 limit 6 to review articles

The 'mp' suffix (see p. 30) automatically gives you a textword search of the title and abstracts, and should give you 241 articles, most of which look very relevant to your question and some of which were missed when you searched MeSH terms alone. While 241 articles (at last count) is a massive set to browse in full, you might like to list them in reverse date order and work backwards from the most recent publication.

Another important strategy for preventing incomplete searches is to use the powerful 'explode' command. The 'explode' function is explained in Problem 2, and you should use it routinely unless you have good reason not to. Try the following search as an example. We are trying to get hold of a good review article about gonococcal arthritis (a rare type of acute arthritis caused by the gonococcus bacterium). Type the MeSH term, with an asterisk for 'focus'

1 *arthritis/

This will give you about 11,400 articles in which arthritis is the focus. Now search for articles on arthritis in which the word 'gonococcal' is mentioned in the title or abstract, by typing

2 gonococcal.tw.

3 1 and 2

This narrows your search drastically to 27 articles, none of which offers a comprehensive overview of the subject. And how many have you missed? The answer is quite a few of them, because the MeSH term 'arthritis' subdivides into several branches, including 'arthritis, infectious'. Try it all again (without erasing the first search), but this time, explode the term 'arthritis' before you start and then limit your set to review articles:

4 exp arthritis/

5 2 and 4

6 limit 5 to review articles

You now have almost 40 articles, including a major overview, [9] which your unexploded search missed. You can demonstrate this by typing

7 6 not 3

which will show you what the exploded search revealed over and above the unexploded one. Incidentally, if you were also thinking of searching under textwords, the syntax for identifying articles about the problem in men would be (**male not female).tw. OR (men not women).tw.**

Problem 6: You don't know where to start searching
Solution: Use the 'permuted index' option.
Let's take the term 'stress'. It comes up a lot but searching for particular types of stress would be laborious, and searching 'stress' as a textword would be too unfocused. We need to know where in the MeSH index the various types of stress lie, and when we see that, we can choose the sort of stress we want to look at. For this, we use the command ptx ('permuted index'). Type

ptx stress

The screen shows many options, including post-traumatic stress disorders, stress fracture, oxidative stress, stress incontinence and so on. This is a useful command when the term you are exploring might be found in several subject areas or contexts.

If your subject word *is* a discrete MeSH term, use the tree command. For example,

tree epilepsy

will show where epilepsy is placed in the MeSH index (as a branch of 'brain diseases'), which itself branches into generalised epilepsy, partial epilepsy, post-traumatic epilepsy and so on.

EXERCISE 5

1 Find where the word 'nursing' might appear as part of a MeSH term.
2 Use the 'tree' command to expand the MeSH term 'diabetes mellitus'.

References

1 Swinglehurst D. Information needs of primary care. *Health Information and Libraries Journal* 2005;**22**:196–204.
2 Jewell D. Approaching the literature. In: Jones R, Kinmonth A-L, eds. *Critical reading for primary care.* Oxford: Oxford University Press, 1995:6–18.
3 Cochrane A. *Effectiveness and efficiency.* London: Nuffield Provincial Hospitals Trust, 1972.
4 Grimshaw J. So what has the Cochrane Collaboration ever done for us? A report card on the first 10 years. *CMAJ* 2004;**171**:747–9.
5 Maynard A, Chalmers I. *Non-random reflections on health services research.* London: BMJ Publishing Group, 1997.
6 Greenhalgh T, Robert G, Macfarlane F, Bate P, Kyriakidou O. Diffusion of innovations in service organisations: systematic literature review and recommendations for future research. *Millbank Q* 2004;**82**:581–629.
7 Russell J, Greenhalgh T, Boynton P, Rigby M. Soft networks for bridging the gap between research and practice: illuminative evaluation of CHAIN. *BMJ* 2004;**328**:1174.
8 Stein K, Allen N. Cross sectional survey of cervical cancer screening in women with learning disability. *BMJ* 1999;**318**:641.
9 Angulo JM, Espinoza LR. Gonococcal arthritis. *Compr Ther* 1999;**25**:155–62.

Chapter 3 **Getting your bearings: what is this paper about?**

3.1 The science of 'trashing' papers

It usually comes as a surprise to students to learn that some (the purists would say up to 99% of) published articles belong in the bin, and should certainly not be used to inform practice. In 1979, Dr Stephen Lock, the editor of the *British Medical Journal* wrote 'Few things are more dispiriting to a medical editor than having to reject a paper based on a good idea but with irremediable flaws in the methods used'. Things have improved since then, but it's not much more than 10 years since Doug Altman claimed that only 1% of medical research is free of flaws. [1] Box 3.1 shows the main flaws that lead to papers being rejected (and which are present to some degree in many that end up published).

Box 3.1 Common reasons why papers are rejected for publication

1 The study did not address an important scientific issue (see Section 3.2).
2 The study was not original – that is, someone else has already done the same or a similar study (see Section 4.1).
3 The study did not actually test the authors' hypothesis (see Section 3.2).
4 A different study design should have been used (see Section 3.3).
5 Practical difficulties (e.g. in recruiting participants) led the authors to compromise on the original study protocol (see Section 4.3).
6 The sample size was too small (see Section 4.6).
7 The study was uncontrolled or inadequately controlled (see Section 4.4).
8 The statistical analysis was incorrect or inappropriate (see Chapter 5).
9 The authors have drawn unjustified conclusions from their data.
10 There is a significant conflict of interest (e.g. one of the authors, or a sponsor, might benefit financially from the publication of the paper and insufficient safeguards were seen to be in place to guard against bias).
11 The paper is so badly written that it is incomprehensible.

Most papers appearing in medical journals these days are presented more or less in standard IMRAD format: Introduction (*why* the authors decided to do this particular piece of research), Methods (*how* they did it, and how they chose to analyse their results), Results (*what* they found) and Discussion (what they think the results *mean*). If you are deciding whether a paper is worth reading, you should do so on the design of the methods section, and not on the interest value of the hypothesis, the nature or potential impact of the results, or the speculation in the discussion.

Conversely, bad science is bad science regardless of whether the study addressed an important clinical issue, whether the results are 'statistically significant' (see Section 5.5), whether things changed in the direction you would have liked them to and whether, if true, the findings promise immeasurable benefits for patients or savings for the health service. Strictly speaking, *if you are going to trash a paper, you should do so before you even look at the results.*

It is much easier to pick holes in other people's work than to do a methodologically perfect piece of research oneself. When I teach critical appraisal, there is usually someone in the group who finds it profoundly discourteous to criticise research projects into which dedicated scientists have put the best years of their lives. On a more pragmatic note, there may be good practical reasons why the authors of the study have not preformed a perfect study, and they know as well as you do that their work would have been more scientifically valid if this or that unforeseen difficulty had not arisen during the course of the study.

Most good scientific journals send papers out to a referee for comments on their scientific validity, originality and importance before deciding whether to print them. This process is known as *peer review*, and much has been written about it.[2] Common defects picked up by referees are listed in Box 3.1.

I once corresponded with an author whose paper I had refereed (anonymously, though I subsequently declared myself) and recommended that it should not be published. On reading my report, he wrote to the editor and admitted he agreed with my opinion. He described 5 years of painstaking and unpaid research done mostly in his spare time and the gradual realisation that he had been testing an important hypothesis with the wrong method. He informed the editor that he was 'withdrawing the paper with a wry smile and a heavy heart', and pointed out several further weaknesses of his study which I and the other referee had missed. He bears us no grudge and, like Kipling's hero, has now stooped to start anew with worn-out tools. His paper remains unpublished, but he is a true (and rare) scientist.

The assessment of methodological quality (critical appraisal) has been covered in detail in many textbooks on evidence-based medicine,[3,4] and in the Users' Guides to the Medical Literature in the *Journal of the American Medical*

Association [5-38]. The structured guides produced by these authors on how to read papers on therapy, diagnosis, screening, prognosis, causation, quality of care, economic analysis, systematic review, qualitative research and so on are regarded by many as the definitive checklists for critical appraisal. Appendix 1 lists some simpler checklists which I have derived from the Users' Guides and the other sources cited at the end of this chapter, together with some ideas of my own. If you are an experienced journal reader, these checklists will be largely self-explanatory. If, however, you still have difficulty getting started when looking at a medical paper, try asking the preliminary questions discussed in Section 3.2.

3.2 Three preliminary questions to get your bearings

Question 1: what was the research question – and why was the study needed?

The introductory sentence of a research paper should state, in a nutshell, what the background to the research is. For example, 'Grommet insertion is a common procedure in children, and it has been suggested that not all operations are clinically necessary'. This statement should be followed by a brief review of the published literature, for example, 'Gupta and Brown's prospective survey of grommet insertions demonstrated that...'. It is irritatingly common for authors to forget to place their research in context since the background to the problem is usually clear as daylight to them by the time they reach the writing-up stage.

Unless it has already been covered in the introduction, the methods section of the paper should state clearly the research question and/or the hypothesis that the authors have decided to test. For example, 'This study aimed to determine whether day case hernia surgery was safer and more acceptable to patients than the standard inpatient procedure'.

You may find that the research question has inadvertently been omitted or, more commonly, that the information is buried somewhere mid-paragraph. While I was writing the third edition of this book, I received a peer reviewer's report on a paper I had submitted to a journal which pointed out that I had not stated my research question. My immediate (and rather cross) reaction was that the research question was surely obvious to scientists in the field. I was unwittingly illustrating the fact that specialist researchers are often so immersed in their own work that they forget to spell out the nuts and bolts for the benefit of their readers.

If the main research hypothesis is presented in the negative (which it usually is), such as 'The addition of metformin to maximal dose sulphonylurea therapy will not improve the control of Type 2 diabetes', it is known as a *null* hypothesis. The authors of a study rarely actually *believe* their null hypothesis when they embark on their research. Being human, they have usually set out to demonstrate a difference between the two arms of their study. But the way scientists do this is to say 'let's *assume* there's no difference; now let's try to disprove that theory'. If you adhere to the teachings of Karl Popper, this *hypotheticodeductive* approach (setting up falsifiable hypotheses which you then proceed to test) is the very essence of the scientific method.[39]

If you have not discovered what the authors' stated (or unstated) research question was by the time you are halfway through the methods section, you may find it in the first paragraph of the discussion. Remember, however, that not all research studies (even good ones) are set up to test a single definitive hypothesis. *Qualitative* research studies, which are as valid and as necessary as the more conventional quantitative studies, aim to look at particular issues in a broad, open-ended way in order to generate (or modify) hypotheses and prioritise areas to investigate. This type of research is discussed further in Chapter 11. Even quantitative research (which the rest of this book is about) is now seen as more than hypothesis testing. As Section 5.5 argues, it is strictly preferable to talk about evaluating the *strength* of evidence around a particular issue than about proving or disproving hypotheses.

Question 2: what was the research design?
First, decide whether the paper describes a primary or secondary study. Primary studies report research first hand, whereas secondary (or *integrative*) studies attempt to summarise and draw conclusions from primary studies. Primary studies (sometimes known as empirical studies) are the stuff of most published research in medical journals, and usually fall into one of three categories:

1 *Experiments* in which a manoeuvre is performed on an animal or a volunteer in artificial and controlled surroundings.
2 *Clinical trials* in which an intervention, such as a drug treatment, is offered to a group of patients who are then followed up to see what happens to them.
3 *Surveys* in which something is measured in a group of patients, health professionals or some other sample of individuals.

The commoner types of clinical trials and surveys are discussed in the later sections of this chapter. Make sure you understand any jargon used in describing the study design (see Table 3.1).[40]

Secondary research is comprised of the following:

1 *Overviews* which are considered in Chapter 8, may be divided into
  a) *(non-systematic) reviews* which summarise primary studies;

b) *systematic reviews* which do this using a rigorous, transparent and auditable (i.e. checkable) method; and

c) *meta-analyses* which integrate the numerical data from more than one study.

2 *Guidelines* which are considered in Chapter 9, draw conclusions from primary studies about how clinicians should be behaving.

3 *Decision analyses* which are not discussed in detail in this book but are covered elsewhere,[41] use the results of primary studies to generate probability trees to be used by both health professionals and patients in making choices about clinical management.

4 *Economic analyses* which are considered in Chapter 10, use the results of primary studies to say whether a particular course of action is a good use of resources.

Question 3: was the research design appropriate to the question?

Examples of the sorts of questions that can reasonably be answered by different types of primary research study are given in the sections that follow. One question that frequently cries out to be asked is this: was a randomised controlled trial (RCT) (see Section 3.3) the best method of testing this particular hypothesis, and if the study was not a randomised controlled trial, should it have been? Before you jump to any conclusions, decide what broad field of research the study covers (see Box 3.2). Once you have done this, ask whether the study design was appropriate to this question. For more help on this task (which some people find difficult until they have got the hang of it) see the Oxford Centre for EBM website (www.cebm.ox.ac.uk) or the journal article by the same group.[42]

3.3 Randomised controlled trials

In a randomised controlled trial (RCT), participants in the trial are randomly allocated by a process equivalent to the flip of a coin to either one intervention (such as a drug treatment) or another (such as placebo treatment). Both groups are followed up for a specified time period and analysed in terms of specific outcomes defined at the outset of the study (e.g. death, heart attack, serum cholesterol level, etc.). Because, *on average*, the groups are identical apart from the intervention, any differences in outcome are, in theory, attributable to the intervention. In reality, however, not every randomised controlled trial is a bowl of cherries.

Some papers that report trials comparing an intervention with a control group are not, in fact, randomised trials at all. The terminology for these

Table 3.1 Terms used to describe design features of clinical research studies

Term	Meaning
Parallel group comparison	Each group receives a different treatment, with both groups being entered at the same time. In this case, results are analysed by comparing groups
Paired (or matched) comparison	Participants receiving different treatments are matched to balance potential confounding variables such as age and sex. Results are analysed in terms of differences between participant pairs
Within-participant comparison	Participants are assessed before and after an intervention and results analysed in terms of within-participant changes
Single blind	Participants did not know which treatment they were receiving
Double blind	Neither did the investigators
Crossover	Each participant received both the intervention and control treatments (in random order), often separated by a *washout* period on no treatment
Placebo controlled	Control participants receive a placebo (inactive pill) which should look and taste the same as the active pill. Placebo (sham) operations may also be used in trials of surgery
Factorial design	A study that permits investigation of the effects (both separately and combined) of more than one independent variable on a given outcome (e.g. a 2 × 2 factorial design tested the effects of placebo, aspirin alone, streptokinase alone, or aspirin + streptokinase in acute heart attack.[40])

is *other controlled clinical trials*, a term used to describe comparative studies in which participants were allocated to intervention or control groups in a non-random manner. This situation may arise, for example, when random allocation would be impossible, impractical or unethical – for example, when patients on ward A receive one diet while those on ward B receive a different diet. (Although this design is inferior to the RCT, it is much easier to execute and was used successfully a century ago to demonstrate the benefit of brown rice over white rice in the treatment of beri-beri.[43]) The problems of non-random allocation are discussed further in Section 4.4 in relation to determining whether the two groups in a trial can reasonably be compared with one another on a statistical level.

Some trials count as a sort of halfway house between true randomised trials and non-randomised trials. In these, randomisation is not done truly at random (e.g. using sequentially numbered sealed envelopes each with a

---

Box 3.2 Broad fields of research

Most quantitative studies are concerned with one or more of the following:

1 *Therapy.* Testing the efficacy of drug treatments, surgical procedures, alternative methods of service delivery or other interventions. Preferred study design is randomised controlled trial (see Section 3.3 and Chapter 6).

2 *Diagnosis.* Demonstrating whether a new diagnostic test is valid (can we trust it?) and reliable (would we get the same results every time?). Preferred study design is cross-sectional survey (see Section 3.6 and Chapter 7).

3 *Screening.* Demonstrating the value of tests which can be applied to large populations and which pick up disease at a pre-symptomatic stage. Preferred study design is cross-sectional survey (see Section 3.6 and Chapter 7).

4 *Prognosis.* Determining what is likely to happen to someone whose disease is picked up at an early stage. Preferred study design is longitudinal survey (see Section 3.6).

5 *Causation.* Determining whether a putative harmful agent, such as environmental pollution, is related to the development of illness. Preferred study design is cohort or case-control study, depending on how rare the disease is (see Sections 3.6 and 3.7), but case reports (see Section 3.8) may also provide crucial information.

6 *Psychometric studies.* Measuring attitudes, beliefs or preferences, often about the nature of illness or its treatment.

Qualitative studies are discussed in Chapter 11.

---

computer-generated random number inside), but by some method which allows the clinician to know which group the patient would be in *before he or she makes a definitive decision to randomise the patient.* This allows subtle biases to creep in, since the clinician might be more (or less) likely to enter a particular patient into the trial if he or she believed that the patient would get active treatment. In particular, patients with more severe disease may be subconsciously withheld from the placebo arm of the trial. Examples of unacceptable methods include randomisation by last digit of date of birth (even numbers to group A; odds to group B), toss of a coin (heads to group A; tails to group B), sequential allocation (patient A to group 1; patient B to group 2, etc.) and date seen in clinic (all patients seen this week to group A; all those seen next week to group 2, etc.).[44]

Listed below are examples of clinical questions which would be best answered by a randomised controlled trial, but note also the examples in

---

Box 3.3 Advantages of the randomised controlled trial design

1 Allows rigorous evaluation of a single variable (e.g. effect of drug treatment versus placebo) in a precisely defined patient group (e.g. post-menopausal women aged 50–60 years).
2 Prospective design (i.e. data are collected on events which happen *after* you decide to do the study).
3 Uses hypotheticodeductive reasoning (i.e. seeks to falsify, rather than confirm, its own hypothesis; see Section 3.2).
4 Potentially eradicates bias by comparing two otherwise identical groups (but see below and Section 4.4).
5 Allows for meta-analysis (combining the numerical results of several similar trials at a later date; see Section 8.3).

---

the later sections of this chapter of situations where other types of study could or must be used instead.

1 Is this drug better than placebo or a different drug for a particular disease?
2 Is a new surgical procedure better than the currently favoured practice?
3 Is a leaflet better than verbal advice in helping patients make informed choices about the treatment options for a particular condition?
4 Will changing from a diet high in saturated fats to one high in polyunsaturated fats significantly affect serum cholesterol levels?

Randomised controlled trials (RCTs) are said to be the gold standard in medical research (Box 3.3). Up to a point, this is true (see Section 3.8), but only for certain types of clinical question (see Box 3.2 and Sections 3.4–3.7). The questions that best lend themselves to the RCT design all relate to *interventions*, and are mainly concerned with therapy or prevention. It should be remembered, however, that even when we are looking at therapeutic interventions, and especially when we are not, there are a number of important disadvantages associated with randomised trials (see Box 3.4).[45,46]

Remember, too, that the results of an RCT may have limited applicability as a result of exclusion criteria (rules about who may not be entered into the study), inclusion bias (selection of trial participants from a group that is unrepresentative of everyone with the condition [see Section 4.2]), refusal (or inability) of certain patient groups to give consent to be included in the trial, analysis of only pre-defined 'objective' endpoints which may exclude important qualitative aspects of the intervention (see Chapter 11) and publication bias (i.e. the selective publication of positive results, often but not always because the organisation that funded the research stands to gain or lose depending on the findings).[47] Furthermore, randomised controlled trials

Box 3.4 Disadvantages of the randomised controlled trial design (see reference 40)

Expensive and time consuming, hence, in practice,

1 many RCTs are either never done, are performed on too few patients or are undertaken for too short a period (see Section 4.6);

2 most RCTs are funded by large research bodies (university or government sponsored) or drug companies, who ultimately dictate the research agenda;

3 surrogate end points are often used in preference to clinical outcome measures (see Section 6.3).

May introduce 'hidden bias', especially through

1 imperfect randomisation (see above);

2 failure to randomise all eligible patients (clinician only offers participation in the trial to patients she or he considers will respond well to the intervention);

3 failure to blind assessors to randomisation status of patients (see Section 4.5).

can be well or badly managed,[48] and, once published, their results are open to distortion by an overenthusiastic scientific community or by a public eager for a new wonder drug.[49] While all these problems might also occur with other trial designs, they may be particularly pertinent when a randomised controlled trial is being sold to you as, methodologically speaking, whiter than white.

There are, in addition, many situations in which RCTs are either unnecessary, impractical or inappropriate:

RCTs are *unnecessary*

1 when a clearly successful intervention for an otherwise fatal condition is discovered;

2 when a previous RCT or meta-analysis has given a definitive result (either positive or negative – see Section 5.5). Some people would argue that it is actually *unethical* to ask patients to be randomised to a clinical trial without first conducting a systematic literature review to see whether the trial needs to be done at all.

RCTs are *impractical*

1 where it would be unethical to seek consent to randomise (see Section 3.9);[50]

2 where the number of participants needed to demonstrate a significant difference between the groups is prohibitively high (see Section 4.6).

RCTs are *inappropriate*

1 where the study is looking at the prognosis of a disease. For this analysis, the appropriate route to best evidence is a longitudinal survey of a properly assembled *inception cohort* (see Section 3.6);

2 where the study is looking at the validity of a diagnostic or screening test. For this analysis, the appropriate route to best evidence is a *cross-sectional survey* of patients clinically suspected of harbouring the relevant disorder (see Section 3.6 and Chapter 7);

3 where the study is looking at a 'quality of care' issue in which the criteria for 'success' have not yet been established. For example, an RCT comparing medical versus surgical methods of abortion might assess 'success' in terms of number of patients achieving complete evacuation, amount of bleeding and pain level. The patients, however, might decide that other aspects of the procedure are important, such as knowing in advance how long the procedure will take, not seeing or feeling the abortus come out and so on. For this analysis, the appropriate route to best evidence is *qualitative research methods* (see Chapter 11).

All these issues have been discussed in great depth by clinical epidemiologists, who remind us that to turn our noses up at the non-randomised trial may indicate scientific naiveté and not, as many people routinely assume, intellectual rigour.[3] Note also that there is now a recommended format, known as CONSORT, for reporting randomised controlled trials in medical journals, which you are now required to follow if you are writing one up yourself.[51] For an in-depth discussion of the pros and cons of the randomised controlled trial, you might like to take a look at the entire issue of the *BMJ* from 31 October 1998 (*BMJ* 1998;317:1167–1261), as well as a book [52] and monograph.[46]

3.4 Cohort studies

In a cohort study, two (or more) groups of people are selected on the basis of differences in their exposure to a particular agent (such as a vaccine, a medicine, or an environmental toxin), and followed up to see how many in each group develop a particular disease or other outcome. The follow-up period in cohort studies is generally measured in years (and sometimes in decades), since that is how long many diseases, especially cancer, take to develop. Note that randomised controlled trials are usually begun on *patients* (people who already have a disease), whereas most cohort studies are begun on *subjects* (or *participants*) who may or may not develop a disease.

A special type of cohort study may also be used to determine the prognosis of a disease (i.e. what is likely to happen to someone who has it). A group of patients who has all been diagnosed as having an early stage of the disease or a positive screening test (see Chapter 7) is assembled (the inception cohort) and followed up on repeated occasions to see the incidence (new cases per year) and time course of different outcomes. (Here is a definition that you should commit to memory if you can: *incidence* is the number of new cases of a disease per year, whereas *prevalence* is the overall proportion of the population who suffer from the disease.)

The world's most famous cohort study, which won its two original authors a knighthood, was undertaken by Sir Austen Bradford Hill, Sir Richard Doll and, latterly, Richard Peto. They followed up 40,000 male British doctors divided into four cohorts (non-smokers, and light, moderate and heavy smokers) using both all-cause (any death) and cause-specific (death from a particular disease) mortality as outcome measures. Publication of their 10-year interim results in 1964,[53] which showed a substantial excess in both lung cancer mortality and all-cause mortality in smokers, with a 'dose–response' relationship (i.e. the more you smoke, the worse your chances of getting lung cancer), went a long way to demonstrating that the link between smoking and ill-health was causal rather than coincidental. The 20-year, [54] 40-year [55] and 50-year [56] results of this momentous study (which achieved an impressive 94% follow-up of those recruited in 1951 and not known to have died) illustrate both the perils of smoking and the strength of evidence that can be obtained from a properly conducted cohort study.

Clinical questions that should be addressed by a cohort study include the following:

1 Does the contraceptive pill 'cause' breast cancer? (Note, once again, that the word 'cause' is a loaded and potentially misleading term. As John Guillebaud has argued in his excellent book 'The Pill', [57] if a thousand women went on the pill tomorrow, some of them would get breast cancer. But some of those would have got it anyway. The question that epidemiologists try to answer through cohort studies is, 'what is the *additional* risk of developing breast cancer which this woman would run by taking the pill, over and above her 'baseline' risk attributable to her own hormonal balance, family history, diet, alcohol intake and so on'?)

2 Does smoking cause lung cancer?

3 Does high blood pressure get better over time?

4 What happens to infants who have been born very prematurely, in terms of subsequent physical development and educational achievement?

3.5 Case-control studies

In a case-control study, patients with a particular disease or condition are identified and 'matched' with controls (patients with some other disease, the general population, neighbours or relatives). Data are then collected (e.g. by searching back through these people's medical records, or by asking them to recall their own history) on past exposure to a possible causal agent for the disease. Like cohort studies, case-control studies are generally concerned with the aetiology of a disease (i.e. what causes it), rather than its treatment. They lie lower down the hierarchy of evidence (see below), but this design is usually the only option when studying rare conditions. An important source of difficulty (and potential bias) in a case-control study is the precise definition of who counts as a 'case', since one misallocated individual may substantially influence the results (see Section 4.4). In addition, such a design cannot demonstrate causality – in other words, the *association* of A with B in a case-control study does not prove that A has *caused* B.

Clinical questions that should be addressed by a case-control study include the following:

- Does the prone sleeping position increase the risk of cot death (sudden infant death syndrome)?
- Does whooping cough vaccine cause brain damage? (see Section 4.4)
- Do overhead power cables cause leukaemia?

3.6 Cross-sectional surveys

We have probably all been asked to take part in a survey, even if it was only a lady in the street asking us which brand of toothpaste we prefer. Surveys conducted by epidemiologists are run along essentially the same lines: a representative sample of participants (or patients) is interviewed, examined or otherwise studied to gain answers to a specific clinical question. In cross-sectional surveys, data are collected at a single time point but may refer retrospectively to health experiences in the past – such as, for example, the study of patients' medical records to see how often their blood pressure has been recorded in the past 5 years.

Clinical questions that should be addressed by a cross-sectional survey include

- What is the 'normal' height of a 3-year-old child? (This, like other questions about the range of normality, can be answered simply by measuring the height of enough healthy 3 year olds. But such an exercise does not answer the related clinical question, 'when should an unusually short child be investigated for disease?' since, as in almost all biological measurements, the physiological [normal] overlaps with the pathological [abnormal]. This problem is discussed further in Section 7.4.)
- What do psychiatric nurses believe about the value of electro-convulsive therapy (ECT) in the treatment of severe depression?

- Is it true that 'half of all cases of diabetes are undiagnosed'? (This an example of the more general question, 'What is the prevalence [proportion of people with the condition] of this disease in this community?' The only way of finding the answer is to do the definitive diagnostic test on a representative sample of the population.)

3.7 Case reports

A case report describes the medical history of a single patient in the form of a story ('Mrs B is a 54-year-old secretary who developed chest pain in June 2005...'). Case reports are often run together to form a *case series*, in which the medical histories of more than one patient with a particular condition are described to illustrate an aspect of the condition, the treatment or, most commonly these days, adverse reaction to treatment.

Although this type of research is traditionally considered to be relatively weak scientific evidence (see Section 3.8), a great deal of information can be conveyed in a case report that would be lost in a clinical trial or survey (see Chapter 11). In addition, case reports are immediately understandable by non-academic clinicians and by the lay public. They can, if necessary, be written up and published within days, which gives them a definite edge over meta-analyses (whose gestation period can run into years) or clinical trials (several months). There are certainly good theoretical grounds for the reinstatement of the humble case report as a useful and valid contribution to medical science, not least because the story is one of the best vehicles for *making sense* of a complex clinical situation.[58] Furthermore, stories are highly memorable (indeed, in most medical schools they are the unit of teaching and learning), but we should not confuse the memorability of a clinical story with its contribution to *research*.[59]

Clinical situations in which a case report or case series is an appropriate type of study include examples as follows:

1 A doctor notices that two babies born in his hospital have absent limbs (phocomelia). Both mothers had taken a new drug (thalidomide) in early pregnancy. The doctor wishes to alert his colleagues worldwide to the possibility of drug-related damage as quickly as possible.[60] (Anyone who thinks 'quick and dirty' case reports are never scientifically justified should remember this example.)

2 A previously healthy patient develops spontaneous bacterial peritonitis – an unusual problem that the average doctor might see once in 10-years. The clinical team looking after her search the literature for research evidence and develop what they believe is an evidence-based management plan. The patient recovers well. The team decides to write this

story up as a lesson for other clinicians – a so-called 'evidence-based case report'.[61]

3.8 The traditional hierarchy of evidence

Standard notation for the relative weight carried by the different types of primary study when making decisions about clinical interventions (the 'hierarchy of evidence') puts them in the following order:[12]

1 Systematic reviews and meta-analyses (see Chapter 8).
2 Randomised controlled trials with definitive results (i.e. confidence intervals which do not overlap the threshold clinically significant effect; see Section 5.5).
3 Randomised controlled trials with non-definitive results (i.e. a point estimate which suggests a clinically significant effect but with confidence intervals overlapping the threshold for this effect; see Section 5.5).
4 Cohort studies.
5 Case-controlled studies.
6 Cross-sectional surveys.
7 Case reports.

The pinnacle of the hierarchy is, quite properly, reserved for secondary research papers, in which all the primary studies on a particular subject have been hunted out and critically appraised according to rigorous criteria (see Chapter 8). Note, however, that not even the most hard-line protagonist of evidence-based medicine would place a sloppy meta-analysis or a randomised controlled trial that was seriously methodologically flawed above a large, well-designed cohort study. And as Chapter 11 shows, many important and valid studies in the field of qualitative research do not feature in this particular hierarchy of evidence at all. In other words, evaluating the potential contribution of a particular study to medical science requires considerably more effort than is needed to check off its basic design against the seven-point scale above. I strongly recommend a recent article in which EBM experts argue for the use of *both* hierarchies of study design *and* common sense judgement when ranking research studies and assessing their relative contribution to a decision.[62]

3.9 A note on ethical considerations

When I was a junior doctor, I got a job in a world-renowned teaching hospital. One of my humble tasks was seeing the geriatric (elderly) patients in casualty. I was soon invited out to lunch by two charming registrars, who (I later realised) were seeking my help with their research. In return for getting my name on the paper, I was to take a rectal biopsy (i.e. cut out a small piece of tissue from the rectum) on any patient over the age of 90 who had constipation. I asked for a copy of the consent form which patients would be asked to sign. When they assured me that the average 90-year-old would hardly notice the procedure, I smelt a rat and refused to co-operate with their project.

I was naïvely unaware of the seriousness of the offence being planned by these doctors. Doing *any* research, particularly that which involves invasive procedures, on vulnerable and sick patients without full consideration of ethical issues is both a criminal offence and potential grounds for a doctor to be 'struck off' the medical register. Getting formal ethical approval for one's research study (see www.corec.ac.uk) and ensuring that the research is properly run and adequately monitored (a set of tasks and responsibilities known as 'research governance'.)[63] can be an enormous bureaucratic hurdle.[64] Ethical issues were, sadly, sometimes ignored in the past in research in babies, the elderly, those with learning difficulties and those unable to protest (e.g. prisoners and the military), leading to some infamous research scandals.[65]

Note, however, that this hand can be overplayed. Research Ethics Committees frequently deem research proposals 'unethical', yet it could be argued that in areas of genuine clinical uncertainty the only ethical option is to allow the informed patient the opportunity to help reduce that uncertainty. Neurologist and researcher Professor Charles Warlow has argued that the overemphasis on 'informed consent' by well-intentioned ethics committees has been the kiss of death to research into head injuries, strokes and other acute brain problems (in which, clearly, the person is in no position to consider the personal pros and cons of taking part in a research study).[66]

These days, most editors routinely refuse to publish research that has not been approved by a Research Ethics Committee, but if you are in doubt about a paper's status, there is nothing to stop you from writing to ask the authors for copies of relevant documents.

References

1 Altman DG. The scandal of poor medical research. *BMJ* 1994;**308**:283–4.
2 Godlee F, Jefferson T. *Peer review in the health sciences*. London: BMJ Publications, 2003.
3 Sackett DL, Haynes RB, Guyatt GH, Tugwell P. *Clinical epidemiology. A basic science for clinical medicine*. Boston: Little Brown & Company, 1991.
4 Sackett DL, Richardson WS, Rosenberg WMC, Haynes RB. *Evidence-based medicine: how to practice and teach EBM*. London: Churchill-Livingstone, 2000.

5 Oxman AD, Sackett DL, Guyatt GH. Users' guides to the medical literature. I. How to get started. Evidence-Based Medicine Working Group. *JAMA* 1993;270: 2093–5.

6 Guyatt GH, Sackett DL, Cook DJ. Users' guides to the medical literature. II. How to use an article about therapy or prevention. A. Are the results of the study valid? Evidence-Based Medicine Working Group. *JAMA* 1993;270:2598–601.

7 Oxman AD, Cook DJ, Guyatt GH. Users' guides to the medical literature. VI. How to use an overview. Evidence-Based Medicine Working Group. *JAMA* 1994;272:1367–71.

8 Laupacis A, Wells G, Richardson WS, Tugwell P. Users' guides to the medical literature. V. How to use an article about prognosis. Evidence-Based Medicine Working Group. *JAMA* 1994;272:234–7.

9 Levine M, Walter S, Lee H, Haines T, Holbrook A, Moyer V. Users' guides to the medical literature. IV. How to use an article about harm. Evidence-Based Medicine Working Group. *JAMA* 1994;271:1615–19.

10 Jaeschke R, Guyatt GH, Sackett DL. Users' guides to the medical literature. III. How to use an article about a diagnostic test. B. What are the results and will they help me in caring for my patients? Evidence-Based Medicine Working Group. *JAMA* 1994;271:703–7.

11 Jaeschke R, Guyatt GH, Sackett DL. Users' guides to the medical literature. III. How to use an article about a diagnostic test. A. Are the results of the study valid? Evidence-Based Medicine Working Group. *JAMA* 1994;271: 389–91.

12 Guyatt GH, Sackett DL, Sinclair JC, Hayward R, Cook DJ, Cook RJ. Users' guides to the medical literature. IX. A method for grading health care recommendations. Evidence-Based Medicine Working Group (published erratum appears in *JAMA* 1996;275(16):1232). *JAMA* 1995;274:1800–4.

13 Wilson MC, Hayward RS, Tunis SR, Bass EB, Guyatt G. Users' guides to the Medical Literature. VIII. How to use clinical practice guidelines. B. what are the recommendations and will they help you in caring for your patients? Evidence-Based Medicine Working Group. *JAMA* 1995;274:1630–2.

14 Hayward RS, Wilson MC, Tunis SR, Bass EB, Guyatt G. Users' guides to the medical literature. VIII. How to use clinical practice guidelines. A. Are the recommendations valid? Evidence-Based Medicine Working Group. *JAMA* 1995;274:570–4.

15 Richardson WS, Detsky AS. Users' guides to the medical literature. VII. How to use a clinical decision analysis. B. What are the results and will they help me in caring for my patients? Evidence-Based Medicine Working Group. *JAMA* 1995;273: 1610–13.

16 Richardson WS, Detsky AS. Users' guides to the medical literature. VII. How to use a clinical decision analysis. A. Are the results of the study valid? Evidence-Based Medicine Working Group. *JAMA* 1995;273:1292–5.

17 Naylor CD, Guyatt GH. Users' guides to the medical literature. XI. How to use an article about a clinical utilization review. Evidence-Based Medicine Working Group. *JAMA* 1996;275:1435–9.

18 Naylor CD, Guyatt GH. Users' guides to the medical literature. X. How to use an article reporting variations in the outcomes of health services. Evidence-Based Medicine Working Group. *JAMA* 1996;**275**:554–8.

19 O'Brien BJ, Heyland D, Richardson WS, Levine M, Drummond MF. Users' guides to the medical literature. XIII. How to use an article on economic analysis of clinical practice. B. What are the results and will they help me in caring for my patients? Evidence-Based Medicine Working Group (published erratum appears in *JAMA* 1997; **278**(13):1064). *JAMA* 1997;**277**:1802–6.

20 Drummond MF, Richardson WS, O'Brien BJ, Levine M, Heyland D. Users' guides to the medical literature. XIII. How to use an article on economic analysis of clinical practice. A. Are the results of the study valid? Evidence-Based Medicine Working Group. *JAMA* 1997;**277**:1552–7.

21 Guyatt GH, Naylor CD, Juniper E, Heyland DK, Jaeschke R, Cook DJ. Users' guides to the medical literature. XII. How to use articles about health-related quality of life. Evidence-Based Medicine Working Group. *JAMA* 1997;**277**:1232–7.

22 Dans AL, Dans LF, Guyatt GH, Richardson S. Users' guides to the medical literature: XIV. How to decide on the applicability of clinical trial results to your patient. Evidence-Based Medicine Working Group. *JAMA* 1998;**279**:545–9.

23 McAlister FA, Laupacis A, Wells GA, Sackett DL. Users' guides to the medical literature: XIX. Applying clinical trial results B. Guidelines for determining whether a drug is exerting (more than) a class effect. *JAMA* 1999;**282**:1371–7.

24 Bucher HC, Guyatt GH, Cook DJ, Holbrook A, McAlister FA. Users' guides to the medical literature: XIX. Applying clinical trial results. A. How to use an article measuring the effect of an intervention on surrogate end points. Evidence-Based Medicine Working Group. *JAMA* 1999;**282**:771–8.

25 Randolph AG, Haynes RB, Wyatt JC, Cook DJ, Guyatt GH. Users' guides to the medical literature: XVIII. How to use an article evaluating the clinical impact of a computer-based clinical decision support system. *JAMA* 1999;**282**:67–74.

26 Barratt A, Irwig L, Glasziou P, Cumming RG, Raffle A, Hicks N *et al.* Users' guides to the medical literature: XVII. How to use guidelines and recommendations about screening. Evidence-Based Medicine Working Group. *JAMA* 1999;**281**:2029–34.

27 Guyatt GH, Sinclair J, Cook DJ, Glasziou P. Users' guides to the medical literature: XVI. How to use a treatment recommendation. Evidence-Based Medicine Working Group and the Cochrane Applicability Methods Working Group. *JAMA* 1999;**281**:1836–43.

28 Richardson WS, Wilson MC, Guyatt GH, Cook DJ, Nishikawa J. Users' guides to the medical literature: XV. How to use an article about disease probability for differential diagnosis. Evidence-Based Medicine Working Group. *JAMA* 1999;**281**:1214–19.

29 Barratt A, Irwig L, Glasziou P, Cumming RG, Raffle A, Hicks N *et al.* Users' guides to the medical literature: XVII. How to use guidelines and recommendations about screening. Evidence-Based Medicine Working Group. *JAMA* 1999;**281**:2029–34.

30 Guyatt GH, Sinclair J, Cook DJ, Glasziou P. Users' guides to the medical literature: XVI. How to use a treatment recommendation. Evidence-Based Medicine Working Group and the Cochrane Applicability Methods Working Group. *JAMA* 1999;**281**:1836–43.

31 Richardson WS, Wilson MC, Guyatt GH, Cook DJ, Nishikawa J. Users' guides to the medical literature: XV. How to use an article about disease probability for differential diagnosis. Evidence-Based Medicine Working Group. *JAMA* 1999;**281**:1214–19.

32 Guyatt GH, Haynes RB, Jaeschke RZ, Cook DJ, Green L, Naylor CD *et al.* Users' guides to the medical literature: XXV. Evidence-based medicine: principles for applying the Users' Guides to patient care. Evidence-Based Medicine Working Group. *JAMA* 2000;**284**:1290–6.

33 Richardson WS, Wilson MC, Williams JWJ, Moyer VA, Naylor CD. Users' guides to the medical literature: XXIV. How to use an article on the clinical manifestations of disease. Evidence-Based Medicine Working Group. *JAMA* 2000;**284**:869–75.

34 Giacomini MK, Cook DJ. Users' guides to the medical literature: XXIII. Qualitative research in health care B. What are the results and how do they help me care for my patients? Evidence-Based Medicine Working Group. *JAMA* 2000;**284**: 478–82.

35 Giacomini MK, Cook DJ. Users' guides to the medical literature: XXIII. Qualitative research in health care A. Are the results of the study valid? Evidence-Based Medicine Working Group. *JAMA* 2000;**284**:357–62.

36 McGinn TG, Guyatt GH, Wyer PC, Naylor CD, Stiell IG, Richardson WS. Users' guides to the medical literature: XXII. How to use articles about clinical decision rules. Evidence-Based Medicine Working Group. *JAMA* 2000;**284**:79–84.

37 McAlister FA, Straus SE, Guyatt GH, Haynes RB. Users' guides to the medical literature: XX. Integrating research evidence with the care of the individual patient. Evidence-Based Medicine Working Group. *JAMA* 2000;**283**:2829–36.

38 Hunt DL, Jaeschke R, McKibbon KA. Users' guides to the medical literature: XXI. Using electronic health information resources in evidence-based practice. Evidence-Based Medicine Working Group. *JAMA* 2000;**283**:1875–9.

39 Popper K. *Conjectures and refutations: the growth of scientific knowledge.* New York: Routledge and Kegan Paul, 1963.

40 Anon. Randomised trial of intravenous streptokinase, aspirin, both, or neither among 17187 cases of suspected acute myocardial infarction: ISIS-2 (ISIS-2 Collaborative Group). Lancet 1988;**ii**:349–60.

41 Dowie J, Elstein A. *Professional judgement: reader in clinical decision making.* Cambridge: Cambridge University Press, 1988.

42 Sackett D, Wennberg JE. *Choosing the best research design for each question. BMJ* 1997;**315**:1636.

43 Fletcher W. Rice and beri-beri: preliminary report of an experiment conducted at the Kuala Lumpur Lunatic Asylum. *Lancet* 1907;**i**:1776–9.

44 Stewart LA, Parmar MKB. Bias in the analysis and reporting of randomized controlled trials. *Int J Technol Assess Health Care* 1996;**12**:264–75.

45 Bero LA, Rennie D. Influences on the quality of published drug studies. *Int J Technol Assess Health Care* 1996;**12**:209–37.

46 Britton A, McKee M, Black N, McPherson K, Sanderson C, Bain C. Choosing between randomised and non-randomised studies: a systematic review. *Health Technol Assess* 1998;**2**:214–18.

47 Landow L. Sponsorship, authorship and accountability. *N Engl J Med* 2002;**346**:290–2.

48 Farrell B. Efficient management of randomised controlled trials: nature or nurture. *BMJ* 1998;**317**:1236–9.

49 McCormack J, Greenhalgh T. Seeing what you want to see in randomised controlled trials: versions and perversions of UKPDS data. United Kingdom prospective diabetes study. *BMJ* 2000;**320**:1720–3.

50 Lumley J, Bastian H. Competing or complementary: ethical considerations and the quality of randomised trials. *Int J Technol Assess Health Care* 1996;**12**:247–63.

51 Altman D. Better reporting of randomised controlled trials: the CONSORT statement. *BMJ* 1996;**313**:570–1.

52 Jadad AR. *Randomised controlled trials: a user's guide.* London: BMJ Publications, 1998.

53 Doll R, Hill AB. Mortality in relation to smoking: ten years' observations on British doctors. *BMJ* 1964;**i**:1399–467.

54 Doll R, Peto R. Mortality in relation to smoking: 20 years' observations on British doctors. *BMJ* 1976;**Ii**:1525–36.

55 Doll R, Peto R, Wheatley K, Gray R. Mortality in relation to smoking: 40 years' observations on male British doctors. *BMJ* 1994;**309**:901–11.

56 Doll R, Peto R, Boreham J, Sutherland I. Mortality in relation to smoking: 50 years' observations on male British doctors. *BMJ* 2004;**328**:1519–28.

57 Guillebaud J. *The Pill and other forms of hormonal contraception: the facts.* Oxford: Oxford university Press, 2004.

58 Macnaughton J. Anecdote in clinical practice. In: Greenhalgh T, Hurwitz B, eds. *Narrative based medicine: dialogue and discourse in clinical practice.* London: BMJ Publications, 1998.

59 Greenhalgh T. Storytelling should be targeted where it is known to have greatest added value. *Med Educ* 2001;**35**:818–19.

60 McBride WG. Thalidomide and congenital abnormalities. *Lancet* 1961;**ii**:1358.

61 Soras-Weiser K, Paul M, Brezis M, Leibovici L. Antibiotic treatment for spontaneous bacterial peritonitis. *BMJ* 2002;**324**:100–2.

62 Atkins D, Best D, Briss PA, Eccles M, Falck-Ytter Y, Flottorp S *et al.* Grading quality of evidence and strength of recommendations. *BMJ* 2004;**328**:1490.

63 Department of Health. *Research governance framework for health and social care.* London: Department of Health, 2001.

64 Wald DS. Bureaucracy of ethics applications. *BMJ* 2004;**329**:282–4.

65 Fairchild AL, Bayer R. Uses and abuses of Tuskegee. *Science* 1999;**284**:919–21.

66 Warlow C. Over-regulation of clinical research: a threat to public health. *Clin Med* 2005;**5**:33–8.

Chapter 4 **Assessing methodological quality**

As I argued in Section 3.1, a paper will sink or swim on the strength of its methods section. This chapter considers five essential questions which should form the basis of your decision to 'bin' it outright (because of fatal methodological flaws), interpret its findings cautiously (because the methods were less than robust) or trust it completely (because you can't fault the methods at all). These five questions – was the study original, whom is it about, was it well designed, was systematic bias avoided (i.e. was the study adequately 'controlled') and was it large enough and continued for long enough to make the results credible – are considered in turn below.

4.1 Was the study original?

There is, in theory, no point in testing a scientific hypothesis that someone else has already proved one way or the other. But in real life, science is seldom so cut and dried. Only a tiny proportion of medical research breaks entirely new ground, and an equally tiny proportion repeats exactly the steps of previous workers. The vast majority of research studies will tell us (if they are methodologically sound) that a particular hypothesis is slightly more or less likely to be correct than it was before we added our piece to the wider jigsaw. Hence, it may be perfectly valid to do a study that is, on the face of it, 'unoriginal'. Indeed, the whole science of meta-analysis depends on there being more than one study in the literature that have addressed the same question in pretty much the same way.

The practical question to ask, then, about a new piece of research, is not 'has anyone ever done a similar study before'?, but 'does this new research add to the literature in any way'? For example,

1 Is this study bigger, continued for longer, or otherwise more substantial than the previous one(s)?
2 Are the methods of this study any more rigorous (in particular, does it address any specific methodological criticisms of previous studies)?

3 Will the numerical results of this study add significantly to a meta-analysis of previous studies?
4 Is the population studied different in any way (e.g. has the study looked at different ethnic groups, ages or gender than previous studies)?
5 Is the clinical issue addressed of sufficient importance, and does there exist sufficient doubt in the minds of the public or key decision makers, to make new evidence 'politically' desirable even when it is not strictly scientifically necessary?

4.2 Whom is the study about?

One of the first papers that ever caught my eye was entitled 'But will it help *my* patients with myocardial infarction'?[1] I don't remember the details of the article, but it opened my eyes to the fact that research on someone else's patients may not have a take-home message for my own practice. This is not mere xenophobia. The main reasons why the participants (Sir Iain Chalmers has argued forcefully against calling them 'patients')[2] in a clinical trial or survey might differ from patients in 'real life' are as follows:

1 they were more, or less, ill than the patients you see;
2 they were from a different ethnic group, or lived a different lifestyle, from your own patients;
3 they received more (or different) attention during the study than you could ever hope to give your patients;
4 unlike most real-life patients they had nothing wrong with them apart from the condition being studied;
5 none of them smoked, drank alcohol or were taking the contraceptive pill.

Hence, before swallowing the results of any paper whole, ask yourself the following questions:

1 *How were the participants recruited?* If you wanted to do a questionnaire survey of the views of users of the hospital casualty department, you could recruit respondents by putting an ad in the local newspaper. However, this method would be a good example of *recruitment bias* since the sample you obtain would be skewed in favour of users who were highly motivated and liked to read newspapers. You would, of course, be better to issue a questionnaire to every user (or to a 1 in 10 sample of users) who turned up on a particular day.
2 *Who was included in the study?* Many trials in the United Kingdom routinely exclude patients with coexisting illness, those who do not speak English, those taking certain other medication and the illiterate. This approach may be scientifically 'clean' but since clinical trial results will be used to guide practice in relation to wider patient groups, it is not

necessarily all that logical.[3] The results of pharmacokinetic studies of new drugs in 23-year-old healthy male volunteers will clearly not be applicable to the average elderly female! This issue, which has been a bugbear of some doctors for some time,[4] has more recently been taken up by the patients themselves, most notably in the plea from patient support groups for a broadening of inclusion criteria in trials of anti-AIDS drugs.[5]

3 *Who was excluded from the study?* For example, a randomised controlled trial may be restricted to patients with moderate or severe forms of a disease such as heart failure – a policy which could lead to false conclusions about the treatment of *mild* heart failure. This has important practical implications when clinical trials performed on hospital outpatients are used to dictate 'best practice' in primary care, where the spectrum of disease is generally milder.

4 *Were the subjects studied in 'real life' circumstances?* For example, were they admitted to hospital purely for observation? Did they receive lengthy and detailed explanations of the potential benefits of the intervention? Were they given the telephone number of a key research worker? Did the company who funded the research provide new equipment that would not be available to the ordinary clinician? These factors would not, of course, invalidate the study itself, but they may cast doubt on the applicability of its findings to your own practice.

4.3 Was the design of the study sensible?

Although the terminology of research trial design can be forbidding, much of what is grandly termed 'critical appraisal' is plain common sense. Personally, I assess the basic design of a clinical trial via two questions:

1 *What specific intervention or other manoeuvre was being considered, and what was it being compared with?* This is one of the most fundamental questions in appraising any paper. It is tempting to take published statements at face value, but remember that authors frequently misrepresent (usually subconsciously rather than deliberately) what they actually did, and overestimate its originality and potential importance. In the examples in Table 4.1, I have used hypothetical statements so as not to cause offence, but they are all based on similar mistakes seen in print.

2 *What outcome was measured, and how?* If you had an incurable disease, for which a pharmaceutical company claimed to have produced a new wonder drug, you would measure the efficacy of the drug in terms of whether it made you live longer (and, perhaps, whether life was *worth* living given your condition and any side effects of the medication). You would not be too interested in the levels of some obscure enzyme in your blood which

the manufacturer assured you were a reliable indicator of your chances of survival. The use of such *surrogate endpoints* is discussed further in Section 6.3.

The measurement of symptomatic (e.g. pain), functional (e.g. mobility), psychological (e.g. anxiety) or social (e.g. inconvenience) effects of an intervention is fraught with even more problems. The methodology of developing, administering and interpreting such 'soft' outcome measures is beyond the scope of this book. But in general, you should always look for evidence in the paper that the outcome measure has been objectively validated – that is, that someone has demonstrated that the scale of anxiety, pain and so on used in this study has previously been shown to measure what it purports to measure, and that changes in this outcome measure adequately reflect changes in the status of the patient. Remember that what is important in the eyes of the doctor may not be valued so highly by the patient, and vice versa.[6]

4.4 Was systematic bias avoided or minimised?

Systematic bias is defined by epidemiologists Geoffrey Rose and David Barker as anything which erroneously influences the conclusions about groups and distorts comparisons.[7] Whether the design of a study is a randomised control trial, a non-randomised comparative trial, a cohort study or a case-control study, the aim should be for the groups being compared to be as like one another as possible except for the particular difference being examined. They should, as far as possible, receive the same explanations, have the same contacts with health professionals and be assessed the same number of times by the same assessors, using the same outcome measures. Different study designs call for different steps to reduce systematic bias.

Randomised controlled trials

In a randomised controlled trial, systematic bias is (in theory) avoided by selecting a sample of participants from a particular population and allocating them randomly to the different groups. Section 3.3 describes some ways in which bias can creep into even this gold standard of clinical trial design, and Figure 4.1 summarises particular sources to check for.

Non-randomised controlled clinical trials

I recently chaired a seminar in which a multidisciplinary group of students from the medical, nursing, pharmacy and allied professions were presenting the results of several in-house research studies. All but one of the studies presented were of comparative, but non-randomised, design – that is, one

Table 4.1 Examples of problematic descriptions in the methods section of a paper

What the authors said	What they should have said (or should have done)	An example of
'We measured how often GPs ask patients whether they smoke'	'We looked in patients' medical records and counted how many had had their smoking status recorded	Assumption that medical records are 100% accurate
'We measured how doctors treat low back pain	'We measured what doctors *say* they do when faced with a patient with low back pain'	Assumption that what doctors say they do reflects what they actually do
'We compared a nicotine-replacement patch with placebo'	'Participants in the intervention group were asked to apply a patch containing 15 mg nicotine twice daily; those in the control group received identical-looking patches'	Failure to state dose of drug or nature of placebo
'We asked 100 teenagers to participate in our survey of sexual attitudes'	'We approached 147 white American teenagers aged 12–18 (85 males) at a summer camp; 100 of them (31 males) agreed to participate'	Failure to give sufficient information about participants. (Note in this example the figures indicate a recruitment bias towards females)
'We randomised patients to either 'individual care plan' or 'usual care'	'The intervention group were offered an individual care plan consisting of…; control patients were offered…	Failure to give sufficient information about intervention (Enough information should be given to allow the study to be repeated by other workers)
'To assess the value of an educational leaflet, we gave the intervention group a leaflet and a telephone helpline number. Controls received neither'	If the study is purely to assess the value of the leaflet, both groups should have got the helpline number	Failure to treat groups equally apart form the specific intervention
'We measured the use of vitamin C in the prevention of the common cold'	A systematic literature search would have found numerous previous studies on this subject (see Section 8.1)	Unoriginal study

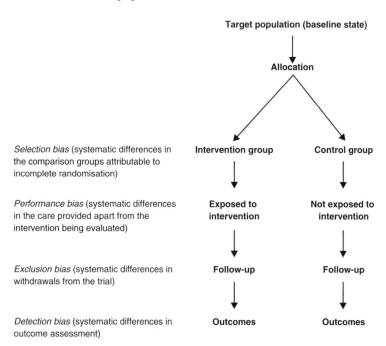

Figure 4.1 Sources of bias to check for in a randomised controlled trial.

group of patients (say, hospital outpatients with asthma) had received one intervention (say, an educational leaflet), while another group (say, patients attending GP surgeries with asthma) had received another intervention (say, group educational sessions). I was surprised how many of the presenters believed that their study was, or was equivalent to, a randomised controlled trial. In other words, these commendably enthusiastic and committed young researchers were blind to the most obvious bias of all: they were comparing two groups that had inherent, self-selected differences even before the intervention was applied (as well as having all the additional potential sources of bias listed in Figure 4.1 for RCTs).

As a general rule, if the paper you are looking at is a non-randomised controlled clinical trial, you must use your common sense to decide if the baseline differences between the intervention and control groups are likely to have been so great as to invalidate any differences ascribed to the effects of the intervention. This is, in fact, almost always the case.[8] Sometimes, the authors of such a paper will list the important features of each group (such as mean age, sex ratio, markers of disease severity and so on) in a table to allow you to compare these differences yourself.

Cohort studies

The selection of a comparable control group is one of the most difficult decisions facing the authors of an observational (cohort or case-control) study. Few, if any, cohort studies, for example, succeed in identifying two groups of subjects who are equal in age, gender mix, socioeconomic status, presence of coexisting illness and so on, with the single difference being their exposure to the agent being studied. In practice, much of the 'controlling' in cohort studies occurs at the analysis stage, where complex statistical adjustment is made for baseline differences in key variables. Unless this is done adequately, statistical tests of probability and confidence intervals (see Section 5.5) will be dangerously misleading.[8,9]

This problem is illustrated by the various cohort studies on the risks and benefits of alcohol, which have consistently demonstrated a 'J-shaped' relationship between alcohol intake and mortality. The best outcome (in terms of premature death) lies with the cohort who are moderate drinkers.[10] Self-confessed teetotallers, it seems, are significantly more likely to die young than the average person who drinks three or four drinks a day.

But can we assume that teetotallers are, *on average*, identical to moderate drinkers except for the amount they drink? We certainly can't. As we all know, the teetotal population includes those who have been ordered to give up alcohol on health grounds ('sick quitters'), those who, for health or other reasons, have cut out a host of additional items from their diet and lifestyle, those from certain religious or ethnic groups which would be under-represented in the other cohorts (notably Muslims and Seventh Day Adventists), and those who drink like fish but choose to lie about it.

The details of how these different features of 'teetotalism' were controlled for by the epidemiologists are discussed elsewhere.[10] In summary, even when due allowance is made in the analysis for potential confounding variables in subjects who describe themselves as non-drinkers, these individuals' increased risk of premature mortality appears to remain.

Case-control studies

In case-control studies (in which, as I explained in Section 3.7, the experiences of individuals with and without a particular disease are analysed retrospectively to identify putative causative events), the process most open to bias is not the assessment of outcome, but the diagnosis of 'caseness' and the decision as to *when* the individual became a case.

A good example of this occurred a few years ago when a legal action was brought against the manufacturers of the whooping cough (pertussis) vaccine, which was alleged to have caused neurological damage in a number of infants.[11] In order to answer the question, 'Did the vaccine cause brain damage'?, a case-control study had been undertaken in which a 'case' was defined as an infant who, previously well, had exhibited fits or other signs suggestive of brain damage within 1 week of receiving the vaccine. A control was an infant of the same age and sex taken from the same immunisation register, who had received immunisation and who may or may not have developed symptoms at some stage.

New onset of features of brain damage in apparently normal babies is extremely rare, but it does happen, and the link with recent immunisation could conceivably be coincidental. Furthermore, heightened public anxiety about the issue could have biased the recall of parents and health professionals so that infants whose neurological symptoms predated, or occurred some time after, the administration of pertussis vaccine might be wrongly classified as cases. The judge in the court case ruled that misclassification of three such infants as 'cases' rather than controls led to the overestimation of the harm attributable to whooping cough vaccine by a factor of three.[11] Although this ruling has subsequently been challenged, the principle stands – that assignment of 'caseness' in a case-control study must be done rigorously and objectively if systematic bias is to be avoided.

4.5 Was assessment 'blind'?

Even the most rigorous attempt to achieve a comparable control group will be a wasted effort if the people who assess outcome (e.g. those who judge whether someone is still clinically in heart failure, or who say whether an x-ray is 'improved' from last time) know which group the patient they are assessing was allocated to. If you believe that the evaluation of clinical signs and the interpretation of diagnostic tests such as ECGs and x-rays is 100% objective, you haven't been in the game very long.

The chapter 'The clinical examination' in Sackett and colleagues' book *'Clinical epidemiology: a basic science for clinical medicine*[12] provides substantial evidence that when examining patients, doctors find what they expect and hope to find. It is rare indeed for two competent clinicians to reach agreement beyond what would be expected by chance in more than two cases in every three for any given aspect of the physical examination or interpretation of any diagnostic test.

The level of agreement beyond chance between two observers can be expressed mathematically as the Kappa score, with a score of 1.0 indicating perfect agreement. Kappa scores for specialists in the field assessing the height of a patient's jugular venous pressure, classifying diabetic retinopathy from retinal photographs and interpreting a mammogram x-ray were, respectively, 0.42, 0.55 and 0.67.[12]

The above digression into clinical disagreement should have persuaded you that efforts to keep assessors 'blind' (or to avoid offence to the visually impaired, *masked*), to the group allocation of their patients are far from superfluous. If, for example, I knew that a patient had been randomised to an active drug to lower blood pressure rather than to a placebo, I might be more likely to recheck a reading which was surprisingly high. This is an example of *performance bias*, which, along with other pitfalls for the unblinded assessor, is listed in Figure 4.1.

An excellent example of controlling for bias by adequate 'blinding' was published in the *Lancet* a few years ago.[13] Azeem Majeed and colleagues performed a randomised controlled trial that demonstrated, in contrast with the findings of several previous studies, that the recovery time (days in hospital, days off work and time to resume full activity) after laparoscopic removal of the gallbladder (the 'keyhole surgery' approach) was no quicker than that associated with traditional open operation. The discrepancy between this trial and its predecessors may have been due to Majeed and colleagues' meticulous attempt to reduce bias (see Figure 4.1). The patients were not randomised until after induction of general anaesthesia. Neither the patients nor their carers were aware of which operation had been done, since all patients left the operating theatre with identical dressings (complete with blood stains!). These findings challenge previous authors to ask themselves whether it was expectation bias (see Section 7.3), rather than swifter recovery, which spurred doctors to discharge the laparoscopic surgery group earlier.

4.6 Were preliminary statistical questions addressed?

As a non-statistician, I tend only to look for three numbers in the methods section of a quantitative paper:

1 the size of the sample
2 the duration of follow-up
3 the completeness of follow-up.

Sample size

One crucial prerequisite before embarking on a clinical trial is to perform a sample size ('power') calculation. In the words of statistician Doug Altman, a trial should be big enough to have a high chance of detecting, as statistically significant, a worthwhile effect if it exists, and thus to be reasonably sure that no benefit exists if it is not found in the trial.[14] If you look up this reference, the nomogram for calculating sample size or power is on p. 456.

In order to calculate sample size, the clinician must decide two things:

1 What level of difference between the two groups would constitute a *clinically significant* effect. Note that this may not be the same as a statistically significant effect. To cite an example from one of the most famous and widely cited clinical trials of all time, you could administer a new drug that lowered blood pressure by around 10 mmHg, and the effect would be a statistically significant lowering of the chances of developing stroke (i.e. the odds are less than 1 in 20 that the reduced incidence occurred by chance).[15] However, if the people being asked to take this drug had only mildly raised blood pressure and no other major risk factors for stroke (i.e. they were relatively young, not diabetic, had normal cholesterol levels and so on), this level of difference would only prevent around one stroke in every 850 patients treated [16] – a clinical difference in risk which many patients would classify as not worth the hassle of taking the tablets.

2 What the mean and the standard deviation (SD; see Section 5.2a) of the principal outcome variable is.

If the outcome in question is an event (such as hysterectomy) rather than a quantity (such as blood pressure), the items of data required are the proportion of people experiencing the event in the population, and an estimate of what might constitute a clinically significant change in that proportion.

Once these items of data have been ascertained, the minimum sample size can be easily computed using standard formulae, nomograms or tables, which may be obtained from published papers,[17] textbooks,[14] free access websites (try http://calculators.stat.ucla.edu/powercalc) or commercial statistical software packages (see e.g. http://www.ncss.com/pass.html). Hence, the researchers can, *before the trial begins*, work out how large a sample they will need in order to have a moderate, high or very high chance of detecting a true difference between the groups. The likelihood of detecting a true difference is known as the *power* of the study. It is common for studies to stipulate a power of between 80% and 90%. Hence, when reading a paper about a randomised controlled trial, you should look for a sentence that reads something like this (which is taken from Majeed and colleagues' cholecystectomy paper described above):

> For a 90% chance of detecting a difference of one night's stay in hospital using the Mann–Whitney U-test [see Table 5.1], 100 patients were needed in each group (assuming SD of 2 nights). This gives a power greater than 90% for detecting a difference in operating times of 15 minutes, assuming a SD of 20 minutes.[13]

If the paper you are reading does not give a sample size calculation *and* it appears to show that there is no difference between the intervention and control arms of the trial, you should extract from the paper (or directly from the authors) the information in (1) and (2) above and do the calculation yourself. Underpowered studies are ubiquitous in the medical literature, usually because the authors found it harder than they anticipated to recruit their participants. Such studies typically lead to a Type II or β error – that is, the erroneous conclusion that an intervention has no effect. (In contrast, the rarer Type I or α error is the conclusion that a difference is significant when in fact it is due to sampling error.)

Duration of follow-up

Even if the sample size itself was adequate, a study must be continued for long enough for the effect of the intervention to be reflected in the outcome variable. If the authors were looking at the effect of a new painkiller on the degree of post-operative pain, their study may only have needed a follow-up period of 48 h. On the other hand, if they were looking at the effect of nutritional supplementation in the preschool years on final adult height, follow-up should have been measured in decades.

Even if the intervention has demonstrated a significant difference between the groups after, say, 6 months, this difference may not be sustained. As many dieters know from bitter experience, strategies to reduce obesity often show dramatic results after 2 or 3 weeks, but if follow-up is continued for a year or more, the unfortunate participants have (more often than not) put most of the weight back on.

Completeness of follow-up

It has been shown repeatedly that participants who withdraw from ('drop out of') research studies are less likely to have taken their tablets as directed, more likely to have missed their interim check-ups, and more likely to have experienced side effects on any medication, than those who do not withdraw.[12] People who fail to complete questionnaires may feel differently about the issue (and probably less strongly) than those who send them back by return of post.[18] People on a weight-reducing programme are more likely to continue coming back if they are actually losing weight.

The reasons why patients withdraw from clinical trials include the following:

1 Incorrect entry of patient into trial (i.e. researcher discovers during the trial that the patient should not have been randomised in the first place because he or she did not fulfil the entry criteria).

2 Suspected adverse reaction to the trial drug. Note that you should never look at the 'adverse reaction' rate in the intervention group without

comparing it with that on placebo. Inert tablets bring people out in a rash surprisingly frequently!

3 Loss of patient motivation ('I don't want to take these tablets any more').
4 Withdrawal by clinician for clinical reasons (e.g. concurrent illness, pregnancy).
5 Loss to follow-up (e.g. patient moves away).
6 Death. Clearly, patients who die will not attend their outpatient appointments, so unless specifically accounted for they might be misclassified as 'drop-outs'. This is one reason why studies with a low follow-up rate (say below 70%) are generally considered invalid.

Simply ignoring everyone who has withdrawn from a clinical trial will bias the results, usually in favour of the intervention. It is, therefore, standard practice to analyse the results of comparative studies on an *intent to treat* basis. This means that all data on patients originally allocated to the intervention arm of the study, including those who withdrew before the trial finished, those who did not take their tablets and even those who subsequently received the control intervention for whatever reason should be analysed along with data on the patients who followed the protocol throughout. Conversely, withdrawals from the placebo arm of the study should be analysed with those who faithfully took their placebo. If you look hard enough in a paper, you will usually find the sentence, 'results were analysed on an intent-to-treat basis', but you should not be reassured until you have checked and confirmed the figures yourself.

There are, in fact, a few situations when intent-to-treat analysis is, rightly, not used. The most common is the *efficacy (or per-protocol) analysis*, which is to explain the effects of the intervention itself, and is therefore of the treatment actually received. But even if the subjects in an efficacy analysis are part of a randomised controlled trial, for the purposes of the analysis they effectively constitute a cohort study (see Section 3.4).

4.7 Summing up

Having worked through the methods section of a paper, you should be able to tell yourself in a short paragraph what sort of study was performed, on how many subjects, where the subjects came from, what treatment or other intervention was offered, how long the follow-up period was (or, if a survey, what the response rate was), and what outcome measure(s) were used. You should also, at this stage, identify what statistical tests, if any, were used to analyse the results (see Chapter 5). If you are clear about these things before reading the rest of the paper, you will find the results easier to understand, interpret and, if appropriate, reject. You should be able to come up with descriptions such as:

> This paper describes an unblinded randomised trial, concerned with therapy, in 267 hospital outpatients aged between 58 and 93 years, in which four-layer compression bandaging was compared with standard single-layer dressings in the management of uncomplicated venous leg ulcers. Follow-up was six months. Percentage healing of the ulcer was measured from baseline in terms of the surface area of a tracing of the wound taken by the district nurse and calculated by a computer scanning device. Results were analysed using the Wilcoxon matched-pairs test.

> This is a questionnaire survey of 963 general practitioners randomly selected from throughout the UK, in which they were asked their year of graduation from medical school and the level at which they would begin treatment for essential hypertension. Response options on the structured questionnaire were '90–99 mm Hg', '100–109 mm Hg', and '110 mm Hg or greater'. Results were analysed using a Chi-squared test on a 3×2 table to see whether the threshold for treating hypertension was related to whether the doctor graduated from medical school before or after 1975.

> This is a case report of a single patient with a suspected fatal adverse drug reaction to the newly-released hypnotic drug Sleepol.

When you have had a little practice in looking at the methods section of research papers along the lines suggested in this chapter, you will find that it is only a short step to start using the checklists in Appendix 1, or the more comprehensive Users' Guides to the Medical Literature referenced in Chapter 3. I will return to many of the issues discussed here in Chapter 6, in relation to evaluating papers on drug trials.

References

1 Mitchell JR. But will it help *my* patients with myocardial infarction? *BMJ* 1982;**285**:1140–8.
2 Chalmers I. What I want from medical researchers when I am a patient. *BMJ* 1997;**310**:1315–18.
3 Bero L, Rennie D. Influences on the quality of published drug studies. *Int J Health Technol Assess* 1996;**12**:209–37.
4 Buyse ME. The case for loose inclusion criteria in clinical trials. *Acta Chir Belg* 1990;**90**:129–31.

5 Phillips AN, Davey Smith G, Johnson MA. Will we ever know how to treat HIV infection? *BMJ* 1996; 313: 608–10.

6 Oliver S, Clarke-Jones L, Rees R, Milne R, Buchanan P, Gabbay G, Gyte G, Oakley A and Stein K. Involving consumers in research and development agenda setting for the NHS: developing and evidence-based approach. *Health Technol Assess* 2004; 18(15): 1–148

7 Rose G, Barker DJP. *Epidemiology for the uninitiated*, 4th edn. London: BMJ Publications, 2003.

8 Britton A, McKee M, Black N, McPherson K, Sanderson C, Bain C. Choosing between randomised and non-randomised studies: a systematic review. *Health Technol Assess* 1998;2:214–18.

9 Brennan P, Croft P. Interpreting the results of observational research: chance is not such a fine thing. *BMJ* 1994;309:727–30.

10 Rimm EB, Williams P, Fosher L, Criqui M, Stampfer MJ. Moderate alcohol intake and lower risk of coronary heart disease: meta-analysis. *BMJ* 1999;319:1523–8.

11 Bowie C. Lessons from the pertussis vaccine trial. *Lancet* 1990;335:397–9.

12 Sackett DL, Haynes RB, Guyatt GH, Tugwell P. *Clinical epidemiology. A basic science for clinical medicine.* Boston: Little Brown & Company, 1991.

13 Majeed AW, Troy G, Nicholl JP, Smythe A, Reed MWR, Stoddard CJ. Randomised, prospective, single-blind comparison of laparoscopic versus small-incision cholecystectomy. *Lancet* 1996;347:989–94.

14 Altman D. *Practical statistics for medical research.* London: Chapman and Hall, 1991.

15 Medical Research Council Working Party. MRC trial of mild hypertension: principal results. *BMJ* 1985;291:97–104.

16 MacMahon S, Rodgers A. The effects of antihypertensive treatment on vascular disease: re-appraisal of the evidence in 1993. *J Vasc Med Biol* 1993;4:265–71.

17 Campbell MJ, Julious SA, Altman DG. Estimating sample sizes for binary, ordered categorical, and continuous outcomes in two group comparisons. *BMJ* 1995;311:1145-8.

18 Boynton PM. A hands on guide to questionnaire research part two: administering, analysing, and reporting your questionnaire. *BMJ* 2004;328:1372–5.

Chapter 5 **Statistics for the non-statistician**

5.1 How can non-statisticians evaluate statistical tests?

In this age where medicine leans increasingly on mathematics, no clinician can afford to leave the statistical aspects of a paper entirely to the 'experts'. If, like me, you believe yourself to be innumerate, remember that you do not need to be able to build a car in order to drive one. What you do need to know about statistical tests is which is the best test to use for common problems. You need to be able to describe *in words* what the test does and in what circumstances it becomes invalid or inappropriate. Box 5.1 shows some frequently used 'tricks of the trade', which all of us need to be alert to (in our own as well as other people's practice).

I have found that one of the easiest ways to impress my colleagues is to let slip a comment such as 'Ah: I see these authors have performed a one-tailed *F*-test. I would have thought a two-tailed test would have been more appropriate in these circumstances'. As you will see from the notes below, you do not need to be able to perform the *F*-test yourself to come up with comments like this, but you do need to understand what its tails mean.

The summary checklist in Appendix 1, explained in detail in the sections below, constitutes my own method for assessing the adequacy of a statistical analysis, which some readers will find too simplistic. If you do, please skip this section and turn either to a more comprehensive presentation for the non-statistician: Sackett's textbook of clinical epidemiology,[1] the 'Basic statistics for clinicians' series in the *Canadian Medical Association Journal*,[2–5] or to a more mainstream statistical textbook.[6] If, on the other hand, you find statistics impossibly difficult, take these points one at a time and return to read the next point only when you feel comfortable with the previous ones. None of the points presupposes a detailed knowledge of the actual calculations involved.

The first question to ask, by the way, is, 'Have the authors used any statistical tests at all'? If they are presenting numbers and claiming that these numbers mean something, without using statistical methods to prove it, they are almost certainly skating on thin ice.

Box 5.1 Ten ways to cheat on statistical tests when writing up results

1 Throw all your data into a computer and report as significant any relationship where '$p < 0.05$' (see Section 5.5a).

2 If baseline differences between the groups favour the intervention group, remember not to adjust for them (see Section 5.2a).

3 Do not test your data to see if they are normally distributed. If you do, you might get stuck with non-parametric tests, which aren't as much fun (see Section 5.2b).

4 Ignore all withdrawals ('dropouts') and non-responders, so the analysis only concerns subjects who fully complied with treatment (see Section 4.6).

5 Always assume that you can plot one set of data against another and calculate an 'r-value' (Pearson correlation coefficient) (see Section 5.4a), and that a 'significant' r-value proves causation (see Section 5.4b).

6 If outliers (points which lie a long way from the others on your graph) are messing up your calculations, just rub them out. But if outliers are helping your case, even if they appear to be spurious results, leave them in (see Section 5.3c).

7 If the confidence intervals of your result overlap zero difference between the groups, leave them out of your report. Better still, mention them briefly in the text but don't draw them in on the graph and ignore them when drawing your conclusions (see Section 5.5b).

8 If the difference between two groups becomes significant $4\frac{1}{2}$ months into a 6-month trial, stop the trial and start writing up. Alternatively if at 6-months the results are 'nearly significant', extend the trial for another 3 weeks (see Section 5.2d).

9 If your results prove uninteresting, ask the computer to go back and see if any particular subgroups behaved differently. You might find that your intervention worked after all in Chinese females aged 52–61 (see Section 5.2d).

10 If analysing your data the way you plan to does not give the result you wanted, run the figures through a selection of other tests (see Section 5.2c).

5.2 Have the authors set the scene correctly?

a) Have they determined whether their groups are comparable, and, if necessary, adjusted for baseline differences?

Most comparative clinical trials include either a table or a paragraph in the text showing the baseline characteristics of the groups being studied (i.e. their characteristics *before* the trial or observational study was begun). Such a table should demonstrate that both the intervention and control groups are similar in terms of age and sex distribution and key prognostic variables (such as the average size of a cancerous lump). If there are important differences in these baseline characteristics, even though these may be due to chance, it can pose a challenge to your interpretation of results. In this situation, you can carry out certain adjustments to try to allow for these differences and hence strengthen your argument. To find out how to make such adjustments, see the section on this topic in Doug Altman's book *Practical statistics for medical research.*[6]

b) What sort of data have they got, and have they used appropriate statistical tests?

Numbers are often used to label the properties of things. We can assign a number to represent our height, weight and so on. For properties like these, the measurements can be treated as actual numbers. We can, for example, calculate the average weight and height of a group of people by averaging the measurements. But consider a different example, in which we use numbers to label the property 'city of origin', where $1 = $ London, $2 = $ Manchester, $3 = $ Birmingham and so on. We could still calculate the average of these numbers for a particular sample of cases but the result would be meaningless. The same would apply if we labelled the property 'liking for x' with $1 = $ not at all, $2 = $ a bit and $3 = $ a lot. Again, we could calculate the 'average liking' but the numerical result would be uninterpretable unless we knew that the difference between 'not at all' and 'a bit' was exactly the same as the difference between 'a bit' and 'a lot'.

All statistical tests are either parametric (i.e. they assume that the data were sampled from a particular form of distribution, such as a normal distribution) or non-parametric (i.e. they do not assume that the data were sampled from a particular type of distribution). In general, parametric tests are more powerful than non-parametric ones and so should be used if at all possible.

Non-parametric tests look at the *rank order* of the values (which one is the smallest, which one comes next and so on) and ignore the absolute differences between them. As you might imagine, statistical significance is more difficult to demonstrate with non-parametric tests, and this tempts researchers to use statistics such as the r value (see Section 5.4a) inappropriately. Not only is the r-value (parametric) easier to calculate than an equivalent non-parametric statistic such as Spearman's σ, but it is also much more likely to give (apparently) significant results. Unfortunately it will also give entirely spurious and misleading estimate of the significance of the result, unless the data are appropriate to the test being used. More examples of parametric tests and their non-parametric equivalents (if present) are given in Table 5.1.

Table 5.1 Some commonly used statistical tests

Parametric test	Example of equivalent non-parametric test	Purpose of test	Example
Two sample (unpaired) t test	Mann–Whitney U-test	Compares two independent samples drawn from the same population	To compare girls' heights with boys' heights
One-sample (paired) t test	Wilcoxon matched-pairs test	Compares two sets of observations on a single sample (tests the hypothesis that the mean difference between two measurements is zero)	To compare weight of infants before and after a feed
One-way analysis of variance using total sum of squares (e.g. F-test)	Analysis of variance by ranks (e.g. Kruskall–Wallis test)	Effectively, a generalisation of the paired t or Wilcoxon matched-pairs test where three or more sets of observations are made on a single sample	To determine whether plasma glucose level is higher 1, 2 or 3 h after a meal
Two-way analysis of variance	Two-way analysis of variance by ranks	As above, but tests the influence (and interaction) of two different covariates	In the above example, to determine if the results differ in males and females
No direct equivalent	χ^2 test	Tests the null hypothesis that the proportions of variables estimated from two (or more) independent samples are the same	To assess whether acceptance into medical school is more likely if the applicant was born in the United Kingdom.
No direct equivalent	McNemar's test	Tests the null hypothesis that the proportions estimated from a paired sample are the same	To compare the sensitivity and specificity of two different diagnostic tests when applied to the same sample
Product moment correlation coefficient (Pearson's r)	Spearman's rank correlation coefficient (σ)	Assesses the strength of the straight-line association between two continuous variables	To assess whether and to what extent plasma HbA1 level is related to plasma triglyceride level in diabetic patients

Table 5.1 Continued

Parametric test	Example of equivalent non-parametric test	Purpose of test	Example
Regression by least-squares method	No direct equivalent	Describes the numerical relation between two quantitative variables, allowing one value to be predicted from the other	To see how peak expiratory flow rate varies with height
Multiple regression by least-squares method	No direct equivalent	Describes the numerical relation between a dependent variable and several predictor variables (covariates)	To determine whether and to what extent a person's age, body fat and sodium intake determine his or her blood pressure

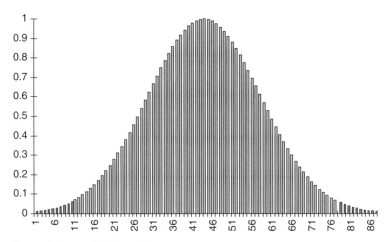

Figure 5.1 Example of normal curve.

Another consideration is the shape of the distribution from which the data were sampled. When I was at school, my class plotted the amount of pocket money received against the number of children receiving this amount. The results formed a histogram the same shape as Figure 5.1 – a 'normal' distribution. (The term 'normal' refers to the shape of the graph and is used because many biological phenomena show this pattern of distribution.) Some

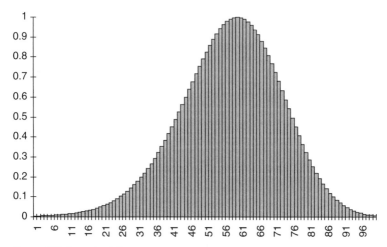

Figure 5.2 Example of skew curve.

biological variables such as body weight show *skew* distribution, as shown in Figure 5.2. (Figure 5.2 in fact shows a negative skew whereas body weight would be positively skewed. The average adult male body weight is 70 kg and people exist who are 140 kg but nobody weighs less than nothing, so the graph cannot possibly be symmetrical.)

Non-normal (skewed) data can sometimes be *transformed* to give a normal-shape graph by plotting the logarithm of the skewed variable or performing some other mathematical transformation (such as square root or reciprocal). Some data, however, cannot be transformed into a smooth pattern, and the significance of this is discussed below. For a further, very readable, discussion about the normal distribution, see Chapter 7 of Martin Bland's book *An introduction to medical statistics.*[12]

Deciding whether data are normally distributed is not an academic exercise, since it will determine what type of statistical tests to use. For example, linear regression (see Section 5.4) will give misleading results unless the points on the scatter graph form a particular distribution about the regression line – that is, the residuals (the perpendicular distance from each point to the line) should themselves be normally distributed. Transforming data to achieve a normal distribution (if this is indeed achievable) is not cheating. It simply ensures that data values are given appropriate emphasis in assessing the overall effect. Using tests based on the normal distribution to analyse non-normally distributed data is very definitely cheating.

c) If the statistical tests in the paper are obscure, why have the authors chosen to use them, and have they included a reference?

There sometimes seems to be an infinite number of possible statistical tests. In fact, most statisticians could survive with a formulary of about a dozen. The rest are small print, and should be reserved for special indications. If the paper you are reading appears to describe a standard set of data that have been collected in a standard way, but the test used is unpronounceable and not listed in a basic statistics textbook, you should smell a rat. The authors should, in such circumstances, state why they have used this test, and give a reference (with page numbers) for a definitive description of it.

d) Have the data been analysed according to the original study protocol?

Even if you are not interested in the statistical justification, common sense should tell you why points 8 and 9 in Box 5.1 amount to serious cheating. If you trawl for long enough you will inevitably find some category of patient which appears to have done particularly well or badly. However, each time you look to see if a particular subgroup is different from the rest you greatly increase the likelihood that you will eventually find one which appears to be so, even though the difference is entirely due to chance.

Similarly, if you play coin toss with someone, no matter how far you fall behind, there will come a time when you are one ahead. Most people would agree that to stop the game then would not be a fair way to play. So it is with research. If you make it inevitable that you will (eventually) get an apparently positive result you will also make it inevitable that you will be misleading yourself about the justice of your case.[7] Terminating an intervention trial prematurely for ethical reasons when participants in one arm are faring particularly badly is different, and is discussed elsewhere.[8]

Going back and raking over your data to look for 'interesting results' (retrospective subgroup analysis or, more colloquially, data dredging) can lead to false conclusions.[8] In an early study on the use of aspirin in the prevention of stroke in predisposed patients, the results showed a significant effect in both sexes combined, and a retrospective subgroup analysis appeared to show that the effect was confined to males.[9] This conclusion led to aspirin being withheld from women for many years until the results of other studies (including a large meta-analysis[10]) showed this subgroup effect to be spurious.

This and other examples are given in a paper by Oxman and Guyatt, 'A consumer's guide to subgroup analysis', which reproduces a useful checklist for deciding whether apparent differences in subgroup response are real.[11]

5.3 Paired data, tails and outliers

a) Were paired tests performed on paired data?

Students often find it difficult to decide whether to use a paired or unpaired statistical test to analyse their data. There is, in fact, no great mystery about this. If you measure something twice on each participant (e.g. lying and standing blood pressure), you will probably be interested not just in the average difference in lying versus standing blood pressure in the entire sample, but in how much each individual's blood pressure changes with position. In this situation, you have what are called 'paired' data, because each measurement beforehand is paired with a measurement afterwards.

In this example, it is having the same person on both occasions which makes the pairings, but there are other possibilities (e.g. any two measurements of bed occupancy made of the same hospital ward). In these situations, it is likely that the two sets of values will be significantly correlated (e.g. my blood pressure next week is likely to be closer to my blood pressure last week than to the blood pressure of a randomly selected adult last week). In other words, we would expect two randomly selected 'paired' values to be closer to each other than two randomly selected 'unpaired' values. Unless we allow for this, by carrying out the appropriate 'paired' sample tests, we can end up with a biased estimate of the significance of our results.

b) Was a two-tailed test performed whenever the effect of an intervention could conceivably be a negative one?

The concept of a test with tails always has me thinking of devils or snakes, which I guess just reflects my aversion to statistics. In fact, the term tail refers to the extremes of the distribution – the dark areas in Figure 5.1. Let's say that this graph represents the diastolic blood pressures of a group of individuals of which a random sample are about to be put on a low-sodium diet. If a low-sodium diet has a significant lowering effect on blood pressure, subsequent blood pressure measurements on these participants would be more likely to lie within the left-hand 'tail' of the graph. Hence we would analyse the data with statistical tests designed to show whether unusually low readings in this patient sample were likely to have arisen by chance.

But on what grounds may we assume that a low-sodium diet could only conceivably put blood pressure down, but could never put it *up*? Even if there are valid physiological reasons why that might be the case in this particular example, it is certainly not good science always to assume that you know the *direction* of the effect which your intervention will have. A new drug intended to relieve nausea might actually exacerbate it, and an educational leaflet intended to reduce anxiety might increase it. Hence, your statistical analysis should, in general, test the hypothesis that either high *or* low values in your data set have arisen by chance. In the language of the statisticians, this means you need a two-tailed test unless you have very convincing evidence that the difference can only be in one direction.

c) Were 'outliers' analysed with both common sense and appropriate statistical adjustments?

Unexpected results may reflect idiosyncrasies in the participant (e.g. unusual metabolism), errors in measurement (e.g. faulty equipment), errors in interpretation (e.g. misreading a meter reading), or errors in calculation (e.g. misplaced decimal points). Only the first of these is a 'real' result which deserves to be included in the analysis. A result which is many orders of magnitude away from the others is less likely to be genuine, but it may be. A few years ago, while doing a research project, I measured a number of different hormone levels in about 30 participants. One participant's growth hormone levels came back about a hundred times higher than everyone else's. I assumed this was a transcription error, so I moved the decimal point two places to the left. Some weeks later, I met the technician who had analysed the specimens and he asked, 'Whatever happened to that chap with acromegaly'?

Statistically correcting for outliers (e.g. to modify their effect on the overall result) is quite a sophisticated statistical manoeuvre. If you are interested, try the relevant section in Doug Altman's book.[6].

5.4 Correlation, regression and causation

a) Has correlation been distinguished from regression, and has the correlation coefficient (r-value) been calculated and interpreted correctly?

For many non-statisticians, the terms 'correlation' and 'regression' are synonymous and refer vaguely to a mental image of a scatter graph with dots sprinkled messily along a diagonal line sprouting from the intercept of the axes. You would be right in assuming that if two things are not correlated, it will be meaningless to attempt a regression. But regression and correlation are both precise statistical terms which serve quite different functions. [12]

The r-value (Pearson's product–moment correlation coefficient) is among the most overused statistical instruments in the book. Strictly speaking, the r-value is not valid unless the following criteria are fulfilled:

1 The data (or, strictly, the population from which the data are drawn) should be normally distributed. If they are not, non-parametric tests of correlation should be used instead (see Table 5.1).

2 The two variables should be structurally independent (i.e. one should not be forced to vary with the other). If they are not, a paired t or other paired test should be used instead.

3 Only a single pair of measurement should be made on each participant, since the measurements made on successive participants need to be statistically independent of each other if we are to end up with unbiased estimates of the population parameters of interest.[13,14]

Every r-value should be accompanied by a p-value, which expresses how likely an association of this strength would be to have arisen by chance (see

Section 5.5a), or a confidence interval, which expresses the range within which the 'true' R-value is likely to lie (see Section 5.5b). (Note that lower case r represents the correlation coefficient of the sample, whereas upper case R represents the correlation coefficient of the entire population.)

Remember, too, that even if the r-value is an appropriate value to calculate from a set of data, it does not tell you whether the relationship, however strong, is causal (see below).

What, then, is regression? The term 'regression' refers to a mathematical *equation* which allows one variable (the *target* variable) to be predicted from another (the *independent* variable). Regression, then, implies a direction of influence, although as Section 5.5 will argue, it does not prove causality. In the case of multiple regression, a far more complex mathematical equation (which, thankfully, usually remains the secret of the computer that calculated it) allows the target variable to be predicted from two or more independent variables (often known as *covariables*).

The simplest regression equation, which you may remember from your schooldays, is $y = a + bx$, where y is the dependent variable (plotted on the vertical axis), x is the independent variable (plotted on the horizontal axis) a is the y-intercept and b is a constant. Not many biological variables can be predicted with such a simple equation. The weight of a group of people, for example, varies with their height, but not in a linear way. I am twice as tall as my son and three times his weight, but although I am four times as tall as my newborn nephew I am much more than six times his weight. Weight, in fact, probably varies more closely with the square of someone's height than with height itself (so that a quadratic rather than a linear regression would probably be more appropriate).

Of course, even when you have fed sufficient height–weight data into a computer for it to calculate the regression equation that best predicts a person's weight from his or her height, your predictions would still be pretty poor since weight and height are not all that closely *correlated*. There are other things that influence weight in addition to height, and we could, to illustrate the principle of multiple regression, enter data on age, sex, daily calorie intake and physical activity level into the computer and ask it how much each of these covariables contributes to the overall equation (or model).

The elementary principles described here, particularly the numbered points mentioned on p. 82, should help you to spot whether correlation and regression are being used correctly in the paper you are reading. A more detailed discussion on the subject can be found in Martin Bland's textbook, [12] and in the fourth article in the 'Basic Statistics for Clinicians' series. [5]

b) Have assumptions been made about the nature and direction of causality?

> **Box 5.2** Tests for causation (see reference 1)
>
> 1 Is there evidence from true experiments in humans?
> 2 Is the association strong?
> 3 Is the association consistent from study to study?
> 4 Is the temporal relationship appropriate (i.e. did the postulated cause precede the postulated effect)?
> 5 Is there a dose–response gradient (i.e. does more of the postulated effect follow more of the postulated cause)?
> 6 Does the association make epidemiological sense?
> 7 Does the association make biological sense?
> 8 Is the association specific?
> 9 Is the association analogous to a previously proven causal association?

Remember the ecological fallacy: just because a town has a large number of unemployed people and a very high crime rate, it does not necessarily follow that the unemployed are committing the crimes! In other words, the presence of an *association* between A and B tells you nothing at all about either the presence or the direction of causality. In order to demonstrate that A has *caused* B (rather than B causing A, or A and B both being caused by C), you need more than a correlation coefficient. Box 5.2 gives some criteria, originally developed by Sir Austin Bradford Hill, which should be met before assuming causality. [13]

5.5 Probability and confidence

a) Have '*p*-values' been calculated and interpreted appropriately?
One of the first values a student of statistics learns to calculate is the *p*-value – that is the probability that any particular outcome would have arisen by chance. Standard scientific practice, which is entirely arbitrary, usually deems a *p*-value of less than one in twenty (expressed as $p < 0.05$, and equivalent to a betting odds of twenty to one) as 'statistically significant', and a *p*-value of less than one in a hundred ($p < 0.01$) as 'statistically highly significant'.

By definition, then, one chance association in twenty (this must be around one major published result per journal issue) will appear to be significant when it isn't, and one in a hundred will appear highly significant when it is really what my children call a 'fluke'. Hence, if you *must* analyse multiple outcomes from your data set, you need to make a correction to try to allow for this (some authors recommend the Bonferoni method [6]).

A result in the statistically significant range ($p < 0.05$ or $p < 0.01$ depending on what you have chosen as the cut-off) suggests that the authors should reject the null hypothesis (i.e. the hypothesis that there is no real difference between two groups). But as I have argued earlier (see Section 4.6), a p-value in the non-significant range tells you that *either* there is no difference between the groups *or* there were too few participants to demonstrate such a difference if it existed. It does not tell you which.

The p-value has a further limitation. Gordon Guyatt and colleagues, in the first article of their 'Basic statistics for clinicians' series on hypothesis testing using p-values, conclude

> Why use a single cut-off point [for statistical significance] when the choice of such a point is arbitrary? Why make the question of whether a treatment is effective a dichotomy (a yes–no decision) when it would be more appropriate to view it as a continuum?[2]

For this, we need confidence intervals, which are considered next.

b) Have confidence intervals been calculated, and do the authors' conclusions reflect them?

A confidence interval, which a good statistician can calculate on the result of just about any statistical test (the t-test, the r-value, the absolute risk reduction (ARR), the number needed to treat and the sensitivity, specificity and other key features of a diagnostic test), allows you to estimate for both 'positive' trials (those which show a statistically significant difference between two arms of the trial) and 'negative' ones (those which appear to show no difference), whether the strength of the evidence is *strong* or *weak* and whether the study is *definitive* (i.e. obviates the need for further similar studies). The calculation of confidence intervals has been covered with great clarity in the classic book *Statistics with confidence*,[15] and their interpretation has been covered by Guyatt and colleagues.[3]

If you repeated the same clinical trial hundreds of times, you would not get exactly the same result each time. But, *on average*, you would establish a particular level of difference (or lack of difference!) between the two arms of the trial. In 90% of the trials the difference between two arms would lie within certain broad limits, and in 95% of the trials it would lie between certain, even broader, limits.

Now, if, as is usually the case, you only conducted one trial, how do you know how close the result is to the 'real' difference between the groups? The answer is you don't. But by calculating, say, the 95% confidence interval around your result, you will be able to say that there is a 95% chance that the 'real' difference lies between these two limits. The sentence to look for in a paper should read something like:

> In a trial of the treatment of heart failure, 33% of the patients randomised to ACE inhibitors died, whereas 38% of those randomised to hydralazine and nitrates died. The point estimate of the difference between the groups [the best single estimate of the benefit in lives saved from the use of an ACE inhibitor] is 5%. The 95% confidence interval around this difference is −1.2% to +12%.

More likely, the results would be expressed in the following shorthand:

> The ACE inhibitor group had a 5% (95% CI −1.2 + 12) higher survival.

In this particular example, the 95% confidence interval overlaps zero difference and, if we were expressing the result as a dichotomy (i.e. is the hypothesis 'proven' or 'disproven'?), we would classify it as a negative trial. Yet as Guyatt and colleagues argue, there *probably* is a real difference, and it *probably* lies closer to 5% than either −1.2% or +12%. A more useful conclusion from these results is that 'all else being equal, an ACE inhibitor is the appropriate choice for patients with heart failure, but that the strength of that inference is weak'. [3]

As Section 8.3 argues, the larger the trial (or the larger the pooled results of several trials), the narrower the confidence interval – and, therefore, the more likely the result is to be definitive.

In interpreting 'negative' trials, one important thing you need to know is 'would a much larger trial be likely to show a significant benefit'?. To answer this question, look at the *upper* 95% confidence interval of the result. There is only one chance in forty (i.e. a $2\frac{1}{2}$% chance, since the other $2\frac{1}{2}$% of extreme results will lie below the *lower* 95% confidence interval) that the real result will be this much or more. Now ask yourself: 'Would this level of difference be *clinically* significant'?, and if it wouldn't, you can classify the trial as not only negative but also definitive. If, on the other hand, the upper 95% confidence interval represented a clinically significant level of difference between the groups, the trial may not only be negative but also non-definitive.

Until fairly recently, the use of confidence intervals was relatively uncommon in medical papers. In one survey of a hundred articles from three top journals (*The New England Journal of Medicine, Annals of Internal Medicine* and *Canadian Medical Association Journal*), only 43% reported any confidence intervals at all, whereas 66% gave a *p*-value. [2] The figure is now considerably higher for journals that follow CONSORT guidelines (see Section 3.3), but even so, many authors do not interpret their confidence intervals correctly. You should check carefully in the discussion section to see whether the authors have correctly concluded (a) whether and to what extent their trial supported their hypothesis, and (b) whether any further studies need to be done.

5.6 The bottom line

Have the authors expressed the effects of an intervention in terms of the likely benefit or harm which an individual patient can expect?

It is all very well to say that a particular intervention produces a 'statistically significant difference' in outcome but if I were being asked to take a new medicine I would want to know how much better my chances would be (in terms of any particular outcome) than they would be if I didn't take it. Four simple calculations (and I promise you they *are* simple: if you can add, subtract, multiply and divide you will be able to follow this section) will enable you to answer this question objectively and in a way which means something to the non-statistician. The calculations are the relative risk reduction, the absolute risk reduction, the number needed to treat and the odds ratio.

To illustrate these concepts, and to persuade you that you need to know about them, let me tell you about a survey which Tom Fahey and his colleagues conducted a few years ago.[14] They wrote to 182 board members of district health authorities in England (all of whom would be in some way responsible for making important health service decisions), and put the following data to them about four different rehabilitation programmes for heart attack victims. They asked which one they would prefer to fund.

Programme A which reduced the rate of deaths by 20%.
Programme B which produced an absolute reduction in deaths of 3%.
Programme C which increased patients' survival rate from 84% to 87%.
Programme D which meant that 31 people needed to enter the programme to avoid one death.

Of the 140 board members who responded, only 3 spotted that all four 'programmes' in fact related to the same set of results. The other 137 all selected one of the programmes in preference to one of the others, thus revealing (as well as their own ignorance) the need for better basic training in epidemiology for health authority board members.

Let's continue with the above example, which Fahey and colleagues reproduced from a study by Salim Yusuf and colleagues.[16] I have expressed the figures as a 2 × 2 table giving details of which treatment the patients received in their randomised trial, and whether they were dead or alive 10 years later.

Treatment	Outcome at 10 years		Total number of patients randomised in each group
	Dead	Alive	
Medical therapy	404	921	1324
CABG	350	974	1325

Simple maths tells you that patients on medical therapy have a 404/1324 = 0.305 or 30% chance of being dead at 10 years. Let's call this risk x. Patients randomised to CABG have a 350/1325 = 0.264 or 26.4% chance of being dead at 10 years. Let's call this risk y.

The relative risk of death – that is, the risk in CABG patients compared with controls – is y/x or 0.264/0.305 = 0.87 (87%).

The relative risk reduction – that is, the amount by which the risk of death is reduced by CABG – is 100% −87%(1 − y/x) = 13%.

The absolute risk reduction (or risk difference) – that is, the absolute amount by which CABG reduces the risk of death at 10 years – is 30.5% −26.4% = 4.1% (0.041).

The number needed to treat – that is, how many patients need a CABG in order to prevent, on average, one death by 10 years – is the reciprocal of the absolute risk reduction (ARR), 1/ARR = 1/0.041 = 24.

The final way of expressing the effect of treatment which I want to introduce here is the odds ratio. Look at the 2 × 2 table presented earlier and you will see that the 'odds' of dying compared to the 'odds' of surviving for patients in the medical treatment group are 404/921 = 0.44, and for patients in the CABG group are 350/974 = 0.36. The *ratio* of these odds will be 0.36/0.44 = 0.82 which is another way of expressing the fact that in this study patients in the CABG group did better.

The general formulae for calculating these 'bottom line' effects of an intervention are reproduced in Appendix 2, and for a discussion on which of these values is most useful in which circumstances, see Jaeschke and colleagues' article in the 'Basic statistics for clinicians' series,[4] or chapter 7 (Deciding on the best therapy) of Sackett *et al.*'s clinical epidemiology textbook.[1]

5.7 Summary

It is possible to be seriously misled by taking the statistical competence (and/or the intellectual honesty) of authors for granted. Statistics can be an intimidating science, and understanding its finer points often calls for expert help. But I hope that this chapter has shown you that the statistics used in most medical research papers can be evaluated by the non-expert using a simple checklist such as that in Appendix 1. In addition, you might like to check the paper you are reading (or writing) against the common errors given in Box 5.2. Finally, if you want pragmatic statistical advice at a slightly higher level than I've given here, check out the website 'Statistics for practical people' on http://www.proaxis.com/~johnbell/sfpp/sfppc.htm

References

1 Sackett DL, Haynes RB, Guyatt GH, Tugwell P. *Clinical epidemiology. A basic science for clinical medicine.* Boston: Little Brown & Company, 1991.
2 Guyatt G, Jaeschke R, Heddle N, Cook D, Shannon H, Walter S. Basic statistics for clinicians: 1. Hypothesis testing. *CMAJ* 1995;**152**:27–32.
3 Guyatt G, Jaeschke R, Heddle N, Cook D, Shannon H, Walter S. Basic statistics for clinicians: 2. Interpreting study results: confidence intervals. *CMAJ* 1995;**152**:169–73.
4 Jaeschke R, Guyatt G, Shannon H, Walter S, Cook D, Heddle N. Basic statistics for clinicians: 3. Assessing the effects of treatment: measures of association. *CMAJ* 1995;**152**:351–7.
5 Guyatt G, Walter S, Shannon H, Cook D, Jaeschke R, Heddle N. Basic statistics for clinicians: 4. Correlation and regression. *CMAJ* 1995;**152**:497–504.
6 Altman D. *Practical statistics for medical research.* London: Chapman & Hall, 1991.
7 Hughes MD, Pocock SJ. Stopping rules and estimation problems in clinical trials. *Stat Med* 1987;**7**:1231–42.
8 Stewart LA, Parmar MKB. Bias in the analysis and reporting of randomized controlled trials. *Int J Technol Assess Health Care* 1996;**12**:264–75.
9 Canadian Cooperative Stroke Group. A randomised trial of aspirin and sulfinpyrazone in threatened stroke. *N Engl J Med* 1978;**299**:53–9.
10 Antiplatelet Triallists Collaboration. Secondary prevention of vascular disease by prolonged antiplatelet treatment. *BMJ* 1988;**296**:320–1.
11 Oxman AD, Guyatt GH. A consumer's guide to subgroup analysis. *Ann Intern Med* 1993;**116**:79–84.
12 Bland M. *An introduction to medical statistics.* Oxford: Oxford University Press, 1987.
13 Bradford Hill A. The environment and disease: association or causation? *Proc R Soc Med* 1965;**58**:295–300.

14 Fahey T, Griffiths S, Peters TJ. Evidence based purchasing: understanding results of clinical trials and systematic reviews. *BMJ* 1995;**311**:1056–9.

15 Gardner M, Altman DG, Bryant T, Machin D. *Statistics with confidence: confidence intervals and statistical guidelines.* London: BMJ Books, 2000.

16 Yusuf S, Zucker D, Peduzzi P, Liher LD, Takaro T, Kennedy WJ *et al.* Effect of coronary artery bypass surgery on survival: overview of ten year results from randomized trials by the coronary artery surgery trailists collaboration. *Lancet* 1994;**344**:563–70.

Chapter 6 **Papers that report drug trials**

6.1 'Evidence' and marketing

If you are a clinical doctor, nurse practitioner or pharmacist (i.e. if you pre-scribe or dispense drugs), the pharmaceutical industry is interested in you and spends a proportion of its multi-million pound annual advertising budget trying to influence you (see Box 6.1). Even if you are a mere patient, the industry can now target you directly through direct-to-consumer advertising (DTCA).[1] When I wrote the first edition of this book in 1995, the stand-ard management of vaginal thrush (candida infection) was for a doctor to prescribe clotrimazole pessaries. By the time the second edition was pub-lished in 2001, these pessaries were available over the counter in pharmacies. Today, clotrimazole is advertised on prime time TV – thankfully after the nine o'clock watershed.

The most effective way of changing the prescribing habits of a clinician is via a personal representative (known to most of us in the United Kingdom as the 'drug rep' and to our North American colleagues as the 'detailer'), who travels a round with a briefcase full of 'evidence' in support of his or her wares.[2] Indeed, as Chapter 12 discusses in more detail, the evidence-based medicine movement has learnt a lot from the drug industry in recent years about changing the behaviour of physicians, and now uses the same soph-isticated techniques of persuasion in what is known as 'academic detailing' of individual health professionals.[3] Interestingly, direct-to-consumer advert-ising often works by harnessing the persuasive power of the patient – who effectively becomes an unpaid 'rep' for the pharmaceutical industry. If you think you'd be able to resist a patient more easily than a real rep, you're probably wrong – a recent randomised controlled trial showed a highly sig-nificant effect of patient power on doctors' prescribing following DTCA for antidepressants.[4]

Before you agree to meet a rep (or a patient armed with material from a newspaper article or DTCA website), remind yourself of some basic rules of research design. As Sections 3.4 and 3.6 argued, questions about the benefits

Box 6.1 Ten tips for the pharmaceutical industry: how to present your product in the best light

1 Think up a plausible physiological mechanism why the drug works, and become slick at presenting it. Preferably, find a surrogate end point which is heavily influenced by the drug, though it may not be strictly valid (see Section 6.2).

2 When designing clinical trials, select a patient population, clinical features and trial length which will reflect the maximum possible response to the drug.

3 If possible, only compare your product with placebos. If you must compare it with a competitor, make sure the latter is given at sub-therapeutic dose.

4 Include the results of pilot studies in the figures for definitive studies, so it looks like more patients have been randomised than is actually the case.

5 Omit mention of any trial which had a fatality or serious adverse drug reaction in the treatment group. If possible, don't publish such studies.

6 Get your graphics department to maximise the visual impact of your message. It helps not to label the axes of graphs or say whether scales are linear or logarithmic. Make sure you do not show individual patient data or confidence intervals.

7 Become master of the hanging comparative ('better' – but better than what?).

8 Invert the standard hierarchy of evidence so that anecdote takes precedence over randomised trials and meta-analyses.

9 Name at least three local opinion leaders who use the drug, and offer 'starter packs' for the doctor to try.

10 Present a 'cost-effectiveness' analysis which shows that your product, even though more expensive than its competitor, 'actually works out cheaper' (see Section 10.1).

of therapy should ideally be addressed with randomised controlled trials. But preliminary questions about pharmacokinetics (i.e. how the drug behaves while it is getting to its site of action), particularly those relating to bioavailability, require a straight dosing experiment in healthy (and, if ethical and practicable, sick) volunteers.

Common (and hopefully trivial) adverse drug reactions may be picked up and their incidence quantified, in the randomised controlled trials undertaken to demonstrate the drug's efficacy. But rare (and usually more serious) adverse drug reactions require both pharmacovigilance surveys (collection of data prospectively on patients receiving a newly licensed drug) and case-control studies (see Section 3.4) to establish association. Ideally, individual rechallenge experiments (where the patient who has had a reaction considered to be caused by the drug is given the drug again in carefully supervised circumstances) should be performed to establish causation.[5]

Pharmaceutical reps do not tell nearly as many lies as they used to (drug marketing has become an altogether more sophisticated science), but they still provide information that is at best selective and at worst overtly biased.[6,7] It often helps their case, for example, to present the results of uncontrolled trials and express them in terms of before-and-after differences in a particular outcome measure.[8] Reference back to Section 3.6 and a look at the classic *Lancet* series on placebo effects,[9–15] or more recent overviews.[16,17] should remind you why uncontrolled before-and-after studies are the stuff of teenage magazines, not hard science.

Dr Andrew Herxheimer, who edited *Drug and Therapeutics Bulletin* for many years, recently undertook a survey of 'references' cited in advertisements for pharmaceutical products in the leading U.K. medical journals. He tells me that a high proportion of such references cite 'data on file', and many more refer to publications written, edited and published entirely by the industry. Evidence from these sources has sometimes (though by no means invariably) been shown to be of lower scientific quality than that which appears in independent, peer-reviewed journals. And let's face it, if you worked for a drug company that had made a major scientific breakthrough you would probably submit your findings to a publication such as the *Lancet* or the *New England Journal of Medicine* before publishing them in-house. In other words, you don't need to 'trash' papers about drug trials *because* of where they have been published, but you do need to look closely at the methods and statistical analysis of such trials.

6.2 Making decisions about therapy

Sackett and colleagues, in their book *Clinical epidemiology. A basic science for clinical medicine*,[5] argue that before starting a patient on a drug, the doctor should

1 identify *for this patient* the ultimate objective of treatment (cure, prevention of recurrence, limitation of functional disability, prevention of later complications, reassurance, palliation, symptomatic relief, etc.);
2 select the *most appropriate* treatment using all available evidence (this includes addressing the question of whether the patient needs to take any drug at all);
3 specify the *treatment target* (how will you know when to stop treatment, change its intensity or switch to some other treatment?).

For example, in the treatment of high blood pressure, the doctor might decide that

1 the *ultimate objective of treatment* is to prevent (further) target organ damage to brain, eye, heart, kidney etc. (and thereby prevent death);

2 the *choice of specific treatment* is between the various classes of antihypertensive drug selected on the basis of randomised, placebo-controlled and comparative trials, as well as between non-drug treatments such as salt restriction; and

3 the *treatment target* might be a Phase V diastolic blood pressure (right arm, sitting) of less than 90 mmHg, or as close to that as tolerable in the face of drug side effects.

If these three steps are not followed (as is often the case – e.g. in terminal care), therapeutic chaos can result. In a veiled slight on surrogate end points, Sackett and his team remind us that the choice of specific therapy should be determined by evidence of what *does* work, and not on what *seems* to work or *ought* to work. 'Today's therapy', they warn (p. 188), 'when derived from biologic facts or uncontrolled clinical experience, may become tomorrow's bad joke'.[5]

6.3 Surrogate end points

I have not included this section solely because it is a particular hobby horse of mine. If you are a practising (and non-academic) clinician, your main contact with published papers may well be through what gets fed to you by a 'drug rep'. The pharmaceutical industry is a slick player at the surrogate end point game, and I make no apology for labouring the point that such outcome measures must be evaluated very carefully.

I will define a surrogate end point as 'a variable which is relatively easily measured and which predicts a rare or distant outcome of either a toxic stimulus (e.g. pollutant) or a therapeutic intervention (e.g. drug, surgical procedure, piece of advice), but which is not itself a direct measure of either harm or clinical benefit'. The growing interest in surrogate end points in medical research reflects two important features of their use:

1 they can considerably reduce the *sample size, duration* and, therefore, *cost* of clinical trials;

2 they can allow treatments to be assessed in situations where the use of primary outcomes would be excessively *invasive* or *unethical*.

In the evaluation of pharmaceutical products, commonly used surrogate end points include

1 pharmacokinetic measurements (e.g. concentration–time curves of a drug or its active metabolite in the bloodstream);

2 *in vitro* (i.e. laboratory) measures such as the mean inhibitory concentration (MIC) of an antimicrobial against a bacterial culture on agar;

3 macroscopic appearance of tissues (e.g. gastric erosion seen at endoscopy);

4 change in levels of (alleged) 'biological markers of disease' (e.g. microalbuminuria in the measurement of diabetic kidney disease);

5 radiological appearance (e.g. shadowing on a chest x-ray).

Surrogate end points have a number of drawbacks. First, a change in the surrogate end point does not itself answer the essential preliminary questions: 'what is the objective of treatment in this patient'? and 'what, according to valid and reliable research studies, is the best available treatment for this condition?' Second, the surrogate end point may not closely reflect the treatment target – in other words, it may not be valid or reliable. Third, the use of a surrogate end point has the same limitations as the use of any other *single* measure of the success or failure of therapy – it ignores all the other measures! Over-reliance on a single surrogate end point as a measure of therapeutic success usually reflects a narrow or naïve clinical perspective.

Finally, surrogate end points are often developed in animal models of disease, since changes in a specific variable can be measured under controlled conditions in a well-defined population. However, extrapolation of these findings to human disease is liable to be invalid:[18,19]

1 In animal studies, the population being studied has fairly uniform biological characteristics and may be genetically inbred.

2 Both the tissue and the disease being studied may vary in important characteristics (e.g. susceptibility to the pathogen, rate of cell replication) from the parallel condition in human subjects.

3 The animals are kept in a controlled environment which minimises the influence of lifestyle variables (e.g. diet, exercise, stress) and concomitant medication.

4 Giving high doses of chemicals to experimental animals may distort the usual metabolic pathways and thereby give misleading results. Animal species best suited to serve as a surrogate for humans vary for different chemicals.

The ideal features of a surrogate end point are shown in Box 6.2 – and microalbuminuria in diabetic kidney disease is probably a good example of a marker that fulfils most if not all of these criteria.[18] If the 'rep' who is trying to persuade you of the value of the drug cannot justify the end points used, you should challenge him or her to produce additional evidence.

One important example of the invalid use of a surrogate end point is the CD4 cell count (a measure of one type of white blood cell which, when I was at medical school, was known as the 'T-helper cell') in monitoring progression

Box 6.2 Ideal features of a surrogate end point

1 The surrogate end point should be reliable, reproducible, clinically available, easily quantifiable, affordable and exhibit a 'dose–response' effect (i.e. the higher the level of the surrogate end point, the greater the probability of disease).

2 It should be a true predictor of disease (or risk of disease) and not merely express exposure to a covariable. The relationship between the surrogate end point and the disease should have a biologically plausible explanation.

3 It should be sensitive – that is, a 'positive' result in the surrogate end point should pick up all or most patients at increased risk of adverse outcome.

4 It should be specific – that is, a 'negative' result should exclude all or most of those without increased risk of adverse outcome.

5 There should be a precise cut-off between normal and abnormal values.

6 It should have an acceptable positive predictive value – that is, a 'positive' result should always or usually mean that the patient thus identified is at increased risk of adverse outcome (see Section 7.2).

7 It should have an acceptable negative predictive value – that is, a 'negative' result should always or usually mean that the patient thus identified is not at increased risk of adverse outcome (see Section 7.2).

8 It should be amenable to quality control monitoring.

9 Changes in the surrogate end point should rapidly and accurately reflect the response to therapy – in particular, levels should normalise in states of remission or cure.

to AIDS in HIV-positive subjects. The CONCORDE trial[20] was a randomised controlled trial comparing early versus late initiation of zidovudine therapy in patients who were HIV positive but clinically asymptomatic. Previous studies had shown that early initiation of therapy led to a slower decline in the CD4 cell count (a variable which had been shown to fall with the progression of AIDS), and it was assumed that a higher CD4 cell count would reflect improved chances of survival.

However, the CONCORDE trial showed that while CD4 cell counts fell more slowly in the treatment group, the 3-year survival rates were identical in the two groups. This experience confirmed a warning issued earlier by authors suspicious of the validity of this end point.[21] Subsequent research in this field attempted to identify a surrogate end point that correlated with real therapeutic benefit – that is, progression of asymptomatic HIV infection to clinical AIDS, and survival time after the onset of AIDS. A review of this work concluded that a combination of several markers (including percentage of CD4 C29 cells, degree of fatigue, age and haemoglobin level) predicts progression much better than the CD4 count.[22]

If you think this is an isolated example of the world's best scientists all barking up the wrong tree in pursuit of a bogus end point, check out the literature on using ventricular premature beats (a minor irregularity of the heartbeat) to predict death from serious heart rhythm disturbance,[23,24] blood levels of antibiotics to predict clinical cure of infection,[25] and the use of the prostate-specific antigen (PSA) test to measure the response to therapy in prostate cancer.[26,27] You might also like to see the fascinating literature on the development of valid and relevant surrogate end points in the important field of cancer prevention(see the entire issue of *Journal of Cellular Biochemistry* 1994;Supplement 19).

Clinicians are increasingly sceptical of arguments for using new drugs, or old drugs in new indications, which are not justified by direct evidence of effectiveness. Before surrogate end points can be used in the marketing of pharmaceuticals, those in the industry must justify the utility of these measures by demonstrating a plausible and consistent link between the end point and the development or progression of disease.

It would be wrong to suggest that the pharmaceutical industry develops surrogate end points with the deliberate intention to mislead the licensing authorities and health professionals. Surrogate end points, as I argued in Section 6.1, have both ethical and economic imperatives. However, the industry does have a vested interest in overstating its case on the strength of these end points, so use caution when you read a paper whose findings are not based on 'hard patient-relevant outcomes'.

6.4 How to get evidence out of a 'drug rep'

Any doctor who has ever given an audience to a 'rep' who is selling a non-steroidal anti-inflammatory drug will recognise the gastric erosion example. The question to ask him or her is not 'what is the incidence of gastric erosion on your drug'?, but 'what is the incidence of potentially life-threatening gastric bleeding'? Other questions to ask 'drug reps', based on an early article in *Drug and Therapeutics Bulletin,*[28] are listed below. For more sophisticated advice on how to debunk sponsored clinical trial reports that attempt to blind you with statistics, see Victor Montori and colleagues' helpful Users' Guide.[29]

1 See representatives only by appointment. Choose to see only those whose product interests you and confine the interview to that product.

2 Take charge of the interview. Do not hear out a rehearsed sales routine but ask directly for the information below.

3 Request independent published evidence from reputable peer-reviewed journals.

4 Do not look at promotional brochures, which often contain unpublished material, misleading graphs and selective quotations.

5 Ignore anecdotal 'evidence' such as the fact that a medical celebrity is prescribing the product.

6 Using the 'STEP' acronym, ask for evidence in four specific areas:

   a) safety – that is, likelihood of long-term or serious side effects caused by the drug (remember that rare but serious adverse reactions to new drugs may be poorly documented);

   b) tolerability, which is best measured by comparing the pooled withdrawal rates between the drug and its most significant competitor;

   c) efficacy, of which the most relevant dimension is how the product compares with your current favourite; and

   d) price, which should take into account indirect as well as direct costs (see Section 10.3).

7 Evaluate the evidence stringently, paying particular attention to the power (sample size) and methodological quality of clinical trials, and the use of surrogate end points. Do not accept theoretical arguments in the drug's favour (e.g. 'longer half-life') without direct evidence that this translates into clinical benefit.

8 Do not accept the newness of a product as an argument for changing to it. Indeed there are good scientific arguments for doing the opposite.

9 Decline to try the product via starter packs or by participating in small-scale, uncontrolled 'research' studies.

10 Record in writing the content of the interview and return to these notes if the rep requests another audience.

References

1 Berndt ER. To inform or persuade? Direct-to-consumer advertising of prescription drugs. *N Engl J Med* 2005;**352**:325–8.

2 Shaughnessy AF, Slawson DC. Pharmaceutical representatives. *BMJ* 1996;**312**:1494.

3 Thomson O'Brien MA, Oxman A, Haynes RB, Davis DA, Freemantle N, Harvey EL. Educational outreach visits: effects on professional practice and health care outcomes. *Cochrane Library* 2000;**2**:CD000409.

4 Kravitz RL, Epstein RM, Feldman MD, Franz CE, Azari R, Wilkes MS *et al*. Influence of patients' requests for direct-to-consumer advertised antidepressants: a randomized controlled trial. *JAMA* 2005;**293**:1995–2002.

5   Sackett DL, Haynes RB, Guyatt GH, Tugwell P. *Clinical epidemiology. A basic science for clinical medicine.* Boston: Little Brown & Company, 1991.

6   Lexchin J. What information do physicians receive from pharmaceutical representatives? *Can Fam Physician* 1997;43:941–5.

7   Roughead EE, Gilbert AL, Harvey KJ. Self-regulatory codes of conduct: are they effective in controlling pharmaceutical representatives' presentations to general medical practitioners? *Int J Health Serv* 1998;28:269–79.

8   Bero LA, Rennie D. Influences on the quality of published drug studies. *Int J Technol Assess Health Care* 1996;12:209–37.

9   Chaput de Saintonge M, Herxheimer A. Harnessing placebo effects in health care. *Lancet* 1994;344:995–8.

10 Thomas KB. The placebo in general practice. *Lancet* 1994;344:1066–7.

11 Johnson AG. Surgery as a placebo. *Lancet* 1994;344:1140–2.

12 Joyce CR. Placebos and complementary medicine. *Lancet* 1994;344:1279–81.

13 Laporte JR, Figueras A. Placebo effects in psychiatry. *Lancet* 1994;344:1206–9.

14 Kleijnen J, de Craen AJ, van Everdingen J, Krol L. Placebo effect in double-blind clinical trials: a review of interactions with medications. *Lancet* 1994;344:1347–9.

15 Gotzsche P. Is there logic in the placebo? *Lancet* 1994;344:925–6.

16 Crow R, Gage H, Hampson S, Hart J, Kimber A, Thomas H. The role of expectancies in the placebo effect and their use in the delivery of health care: a systematic review. *Health Technol Assess* 1999;3(3):1–96.

17 Macedo A, Farre M, Banos JE. Placebo effect and placebos: what are we talking about? Some conceptual and historical considerations. *Eur J Clin Pharmacol* 2003;59:337–42.

18 Gotzsche PC, Liberati A, Torri V, Rossetti L. Beware of surrogate outcome measures. *Int J Technol Assess Health Care* 1996;12:238–46.

19 Kimbrough RD. Determining acceptable risks: experimental and epidemiological issues. *Clin Chem* 1994;40:1448–53.

20 Concorde: MRC/ANRS randomised double-blind controlled trial of immediate and deferred zidovudine in symptom-free HIV infection. Concorde Coordinating Committee. *Lancet* 1994;343:871–81.

21 Jacobson MA, Bacchetti P, Kolokathis A, Chaisson RE, Szabo S, Polsky B *et al.* Surrogate markers for survival in patients with AIDS and AIDS related complex treated with zidovudine. *BMJ* 1991;302:73–8.

22 Hughes MD, Daniels MJ, Fischl MA, Kim S, Schooley RT. CD4 cell count as a surrogate endpoint in HIV clinical trials: a meta-analysis of studies of the AIDS Clinical Trials Group. *AIDS* 1998;12:1823–32.

23 Epstein AE, Hallstrom AP, Rogers WJ, Liebson PR, Seals AA, Anderson JL *et al.* Mortality following ventricular arrhythmia suppression by encainide, flecainide, and moricizine after myocardial infarction. The original design concept of the Cardiac Arrhythmia Suppression Trial (CAST). *JAMA* 1993;270:2451–5.

24 Lipicky RJ, Packer M. Role of surrogate end points in the evaluation of drugs for heart failure. *J Am Coll Cardiol* 1993;22:179A–84A.

25 Hyatt JM, McKinnon PS, Zimmer GS, Schentag JJ. The importance of pharma-cokinetic/pharmacodynamic surrogate markers to outcome. Focus on antibacterial agents. *Clin Pharmacokinet* 1995;**28**:143–60.

26 Carducci MA, DeWeese TL, Nelson JB. Prostate-specific antigen and other markers of therapeutic response. *Urol Clin North Am* 1999;**26**:291–302, viii.

27 Schroder FH, Kranse R, Barbet N, Hop WC, Kandra A, Lassus M. Prostate-specific antigen: a surrogate endpoint for screening new agents against prostate cancer? *Prostate* 2000;**42**:107–15.

28 Anonymous. Getting good value from drug reps. *Drug Ther Bull* 1983;**21**:13–15.

29 Montori VM, Jaeschke R, Schunemann HJ, Bhandari M, Brozek JL, Devereaux PJ *et al.* Users' guide to detecting misleading claims in clinical research reports. *BMJ* 2004;**329**:1093–6.

Chapter 7 **Papers that report diagnostic or screening tests**

7.1 Ten men in the dock

If you are new to the concept of validating diagnostic tests, and if algebraic explanations ('let's call this value *x*...') leave you cold, the following example may help you. Ten men are awaiting trial for murder. Only three of them actually committed a murder; the other seven are innocent of any crime. A jury hears each case and finds six of the men guilty of murder. Two of the convicted are true murderers. Four men are wrongly imprisoned. One murderer walks free.

This information can be expressed in what is known as a 2 × 2 table (Figure 7.1). Note that the 'truth' (i.e. whether or not the men really committed a murder) is expressed along the horizontal title row, whereas the jury's verdict (which may or may not reflect the truth) is expressed down the vertical title row.

You should be able to see that these figures, if they are typical, reflect a number of features of this particular jury:

1 the jury correctly identifies two in every three true murderers;
2 it correctly acquits three out of every seven innocent people;
3 if this jury has found a person guilty, there is still only a one in three chance that he or she is actually a murderer;
4 if this jury found a person innocent, he has a three in four chance of actually being innocent; and
5 in 5 cases out of every 10 the jury gets the verdict right.

These five features constitute, respectively, the sensitivity, specificity, positive predictive value, negative predictive value and accuracy of this jury's performance. The rest of this chapter considers these five features applied to diagnostic (or screening) tests when compared with a 'true' diagnosis or gold standard. Section 7.4 also introduces a sixth, slightly more complicated (but very useful), feature of a diagnostic test – the likelihood ratio. (After you have read the rest of this chapter, look back at this section. You should, by then,

		True criminal status	
		Murderer	Not murderer
Jury verdict	'Guilty'	Rightly convicted **2 men**	Wrongly convicted **4 men**
	'Innocent'	**1 man** Wrongly acquitted	**3 men** Rightly acquitted

Figure 7.1 2 × 2 table showing outcome of trial for ten men accused of murder.

be able to work out that the likelihood ratio of a positive jury verdict in the above example is 1.17, and that of a negative one 0.78. If you can't, don't worry – many eminent clinicians have no idea what a likelihood ratio is.)

7.2 Validating diagnostic tests against a gold standard

Our window cleaner told me the other day that he had been feeling thirsty recently and had asked his general practitioner to be tested for diabetes, which runs in his family. The nurse in his general practitioner's surgery had asked him to produce a urine specimen and dipped a special stick in it. The stick stayed green, which meant, apparently, that there was no sugar (glucose) in his urine. This, the nurse had said, meant that he did not have diabetes.

I had trouble explaining to the window cleaner that the test result did not necessarily mean this at all, any more than a guilty verdict *necessarily* makes someone a murderer. The definition of diabetes, according to the World Health Organisation, is a blood glucose level above 7 mmol/l in the fasting state, or above 11.1 mmol/l 2 h after a 100 g oral glucose load (the much-dreaded 'glucose tolerance test', where the participant has to glug down every last drop of a sickly glucose drink and wait 2 h for a blood test). These values must be achieved on two separate occasions if the person has no symptoms, but on only one occasion if they have typical symptoms of diabetes (thirst, passing large amounts of urine and so on).

These stringent criteria can be termed the *gold standard* for diagnosing diabetes. In other words, if you fulfil the WHO criteria you can call yourself diabetic, and if you don't, you can't (although note that experts rightly challenge categorical statements such as this – and indeed, since the first edition of this book was published the cut-off values in the 'gold standard' test for diabetes using blood glucose levels have all changed).[1] The same cannot be

		Result of gold standard test	
		Disease positive **a + c**	Disease negative **b + d**
Result of screening test	Test positive **a + b**	True positive **a**	False positive **b**
	c + d	**c**	**d**
	Test negative	False negative	True negative

Figure 7.2 2 × 2 table notation for expressing the results of a validation study for a diagnostic or screening test.

said for dipping a stick into a random urine specimen. For one thing, you might be a true diabetic but have a high renal threshold – that is, your kidneys conserve glucose much better than most people's, so your blood glucose level would have to be much higher than most people's for any glucose to appear in your urine. Alternatively, you may be an otherwise normal individual with a *low* renal threshold, so glucose leaks into your urine even when there isn't any excess in your blood. In fact, as anyone with diabetes will tell you, diabetes is very often associated with a negative test for urine glucose.

There are, however, many advantages in using a urine dipstick rather than the full-blown glucose tolerance test to 'screen' people for diabetes. The test is cheap, convenient, easy to perform and interpret, acceptable to patients and gives an instant yes/no result. In real life, people like my window cleaner may decline to take an oral glucose tolerance test. Even if he was prepared to go ahead with it, his general practitioner might decide that the window cleaner's symptoms did not merit the expense of this relatively sophisticated investigation. I hope you can see that even though the urine test cannot say for sure if someone is diabetic, it has a definite practical edge over the gold standard. That, of course, is why people use it!

In order to assess objectively just how useful the urine glucose test for diabetes is, we would need to select a sample of people (say 100) and do two tests on each of them: the urine test (screening test) and a standard glucose tolerance test (gold standard). We could then see, for each person, whether the result of the screening test matched the gold standard. Such an exercise is known as a *validation study*. We could express the results of the validation study in a 2 × 2 table (also known as a 2 × 2 matrix) as in Figure 7.2, and calculate various features of the test as in Table 7.1, just as we did for the features of the jury in Section 7.1.

Table 7.1 Features of a diagnostic test which can be calculated by comparing it with a gold standard in a validation study

Feature of the test	Alternative name	Question which the feature addresses	Formula (see Figure 7.1)
Sensitivity	True positive rate (*Positive in Disease*)	How good is this test at picking up people who have the condition?	$a/a + c$
Specificity	True negative rate (*Negative in Health*)	How good is this test at correctly excluding people without the condition?	$d/b + d$
Positive predictive value (PPV)	Post-test probability of a positive test	If a person tests positive, what is the probability that (s)he has the condition?	$a/a + b$
Negative predictive value (NPV)	Indicates the post-test probability of a negative test*	If a person tests negative, what is the probability that (s)he does not have the condition?	$d/c + d$
Accuracy	—	What proportion of all tests have given the correct result (i.e. true positives and true negatives as a proportion of all results)?	$a + d/ a + b + c + d$
Likelihood ratio of a positive test	—	How much more likely is positive test to be found in a person with, as opposed to without, the condition?	Sensitivity/ $(1 -$ specificity)

*The post-test probability of a negative test is $(1 -$ NPV).

If the values for the various features of a test (such as sensitivity and specificity) fell within reasonable limits, we would be able to say that the test was *valid* (see Question 7 below). The validity of urine testing for glucose in diagnosing diabetes has been looked at by Andersson and colleagues,[2] whose data I have used in the example in Figure 7.3. In fact, the original study was performed on 3268 participants, of whom 67 either refused to produce a specimen or, for some other reason, were not adequately tested. For simplicity's sake, I have ignored these irregularities and expressed the results in terms of a denominator (total number tested) of 1000 participants.

In actual fact, these data came from an epidemiological survey to detect the prevalence of diabetes in a population; the validation of urine testing was a side issue to the main study. If the validation had been the main aim of the study, the participants selected would have included far more diabetic

		Result of glucose tolerance test	
		Diabetes positive 27 subjects	Diabetes negative 973 subjects
Result of urine test for glucose	Glucose present	True positive	False positive
	13 subjects	6	7
	987 subjects	21	966
	Glucose absent	False negative	True negative

Figure 7.3 2 × 2 table showing results of validation study of urine glucose testing for diabetes against gold standard of glucose tolerance test (based on Andersson *et al.*).[2]

individuals, as Question 2 in Section 7.3 will show. If you look up the original paper, you will also find that the gold standard for diagnosing true diabetes was not the oral glucose tolerance test but a more unconventional series of observations. Nevertheless, the example serves its purpose, since it provides us with some figures to put through the equations listed in the last column of Table 7.1. We can calculate the important features of the urine test for diabetes as follows:

- Sensitivity $= a/a + c = 6/27 = 22.2\%$
- Specificity $= d/b + d = 966/973 = 99.3\%$
- Positive predictive value $= a/a + b = 6/13 = 46.2\%$
- Negative predictive value $= d/c + d = 966/987 = 97.9\%$
- Accuracy $= (a + d)/(a + b + c + d) = 972/1000 = 97.2\%$
- Likelihood ratio of a positive test $=$ Sensitivity$/(1 -$ specificity$) = 22.2/0.7 = 32$
- Likelihood ratio of a negative test $= (1 -$ sensitivity$)/$specificity $= 77.8/99.3 = 0.78$

From these features, you can probably see why I did not share the window cleaner's assurance that he did not have diabetes. A positive urine glucose test is only 22% sensitive, which means that the test misses nearly four-fifths of true diabetics. In the presence of classical symptoms and a family history, the window cleaner's baseline odds (pre-test likelihood) of having the condition are pretty high, and they are only reduced to about four-fifths of this (the negative likelihood ratio, 0.78; see Section 7.4) after a single negative urine test. In view of his symptoms, this man clearly needs to undergo a more definitive test for diabetes.[3] Note that as the definitions in Table 7.1 show, if the test had been positive the window cleaner would have good reason to be concerned, since even though the test is not very *sensitive* (i.e. it is not good at picking up people with the disease), it is pretty *specific* (i.e. it *is* good at excluding people without the disease).

Students often get mixed up about the sensitivity/specificity dimension of a test and the positive/negative predictive value dimension. As a rule of thumb, the sensitivity or specificity tells you about the *test in general*, whereas the predictive value tells you about *what a particular test result means for the patient in front of you*. Hence, sensitivity and specificity are generally used more by epidemiologists and public health specialists whose day-to-day work involves making decisions about *populations*.

A screening mammogram (breast x-ray) might have an 80% sensitivity and a 90% specificity for detecting breast cancer, which means that the test will pick up 80% of cancers and exclude 90% of women without cancer. But imagine you were a GP or practice nurse and a patient comes to see you for the result of her mammogram. The question she will want answered is (if the test has come back positive), 'What is the chance that I've got cancer'? or (if it has come back negative) 'What is the chance that I can now forget about the possibility of cancer'? Many patients (and far too many health professionals) assume that the negative predictive value of a test is 100% – that is, if the test is 'normal' or 'clear' they think there is no chance of the disease being present – and you only need to read the confessional stories in women's magazines ('I was told I had cancer but tests later proved the doctors wrong') to find examples of women who have assumed that the positive predictive value of a test is 100%.

7.3 Ten questions to ask about a paper which claims to validate a diagnostic or screening test

In preparing the tips below, I have drawn on three main published sources: the Users' Guides to the Medical Literature[4,5] and the book by the same authors;[6] a more recent article in the *Journal of the American Medical Association*,[7] and David Mant's simple and pragmatic guidelines for 'testing a test'.[8] Like many of the checklists in this book, these are no more than pragmatic rules of thumb for the novice critical appraiser: for a much more comprehensive and rigorously developed set of criteria (which has the downside of running to 234 pages) known as the QADAS (Quality in Diagnostic and Screening tests) checklist, see a recent review by the UK Health Technology Assessment Programme.[9]

Question 1: is this test potentially relevant to my practice?
This is the 'so what'? question which Sackett and colleagues call the *utility* of the test[6]. Even if this test were 100% valid, accurate and reliable, would it help me? Would it identify a treatable disorder? If so, would I use it in

preference to the test I use now? Could I (or my patients or the taxpayer) afford it? Would my patients consent to it? Would it change the probabilities for competing diagnoses sufficiently for me to alter my treatment plan? If the answers to these questions are all 'no', you may be able to reject the paper without reading further than the abstract or introduction.

Question 2: has the test been compared with a true gold standard?

You need to ask, first, whether the test has been compared with anything at all! Papers have occasionally been written (and, in the past, published) in which nothing has been done except perform the new test on a few dozen participants. This exercise may give a range of possible results for the test, but it certainly does not confirm that the 'high' results indicate that target disorder (the disease you are looking for) is present or that the 'low' results indicate that it isn't.

Next, you should verify that the 'gold standard' test used in the survey merits the term. A good way of assessing a gold standard is to use the 'so what?' questions listed above. For many conditions, there is no absolute gold standard diagnostic test which will say for certain whether it is present or not. Unsurprisingly, these tend to be the very conditions for which new tests are most actively sought! Hence, the authors of such papers may need to develop and justify a combination of criteria against which the new test is to be assessed. One specific point to check is that the test being validated here (or a variant of it) is not being used to contribute to the definition of the gold standard.

Question 3: did this validation study include an appropriate spectrum of participants?

If you validated a new test for cholesterol in 100 healthy male medical students, you would not be able to say how the test would perform in women, children, older people, those with diseases that seriously raise the cholesterol level, or even those who had never been to medical school! Although few people would be naïve enough to select quite such a biased sample for their validation study, one paper found that only 27% of published studies explicitly defined the spectrum of participants tested in terms of age, sex, symptoms and/or disease severity, and specific eligibility criteria.[8]

Defining both the range of participants and the spectrum of disease to be included is essential if the values for the different features of the test are to be worth quoting – that is, if they are to be transferable to other settings. A particular diagnostic test may, conceivably, be more sensitive in female participants than males, or in younger rather than older participants. For the same reasons, as Sackett and colleagues stipulate, the participants on which any test is verified should include those with both mild and severe disease, treated and untreated, and those with different but commonly confused conditions.[6]

While the sensitivity and specificity of a test are virtually constant whatever the prevalence of the condition, the positive and negative predictive values are crucially dependent on prevalence. This is why general practitioners are, often rightly, sceptical of the utility of tests developed exclusively in a secondary care population, where the severity of disease tends to be greater (see Section 4.2), and why a good *diagnostic* test (generally used when the patient has some symptoms suggestive of the disease in question) is not necessarily a good *screening* test (generally used in people without symptoms, who are drawn from a population with a much lower prevalence of the disease).

Question 4: has workup bias been avoided?

This is easy to check. It simply means, 'did everyone who got the new diagnostic test also get the gold standard, and vice versa'? I hope you have no problem spotting the potential bias in studies where the gold standard test is only performed on people who have already tested positive for the test being validated. There are, in addition, a number of more subtle aspects of workup bias which are beyond the scope of this book. If you are interested, you could follow the discussion on this subject in Reid and colleagues' paper.[7]

Question 5: has expectation bias been avoided?

Expectation bias occurs when pathologists and others who interpret diagnostic specimens are subconsciously influenced by the knowledge of the particular features of the case – for example, the presence of chest pain when interpreting an ECG. In the context of validating diagnostic tests against a gold standard, the question means, 'did the people who interpreted one of the tests know what result the other test had shown on each particular participant?' As I explained in Section 4.5, all assessments should be 'blind' – that is, the person interpreting the test should not be given any inkling of what the result is expected to be in any particular case.

Question 6: was the test shown to be reproducible both within and between observers?

If the same observer performs the same test on two occasions on a participant whose characteristics have not changed, they will get different results in a proportion of cases. All tests show this feature to some extent, but a test with a reproducibility of 99% is clearly in a different league from one with a reproducibility of 50%. A number of factors which may contribute to the poor reproducibility of a diagnostic test: the technical precision of the equipment, observer variability (e.g. in comparing a colour with a reference chart), arithmetical errors and so on.

Look back again at Section 4.5 to remind yourself of the problem of interobserver agreement. Given the same result to interpret, two people will agree in only a proportion of cases, generally expressed as the Kappa score. If the test in question gives results in terms of numbers (such as the blood cholesterol level in mmol/l), inter-observer agreement is hardly an issue. If, however, the test involves reading x-rays (such as the mammogram example in Section 4.5) or asking a person questions about their drinking habits,[10] it is important to confirm that reproducibility between observers is at an acceptable level.

Question 7: what are the features of the test as derived from this validation study?

All the above standards could have been met, but the test might still be worthless because the test itself is not valid – that is, its sensitivity, specificity and other crucial features are too low. This is arguably the case for using urine glucose as a screening test for diabetes (see Section 7.2 above). After all, if a test has a false negative rate of nearly 80%, it is more likely to mislead the clinician than assist the diagnosis if the target disorder is actually present.

There are no absolutes for the validity of a screening test, since what counts as acceptable depends on the condition being screened for. Few of us would quibble about a test for colour blindness that was 95% sensitive and 80% specific, but nobody ever died of colour blindness. The Guthrie heel-prick screening test for congenital hypothyroidism, performed on all babies in the United Kingdom soon after birth, is over 99% sensitive but has a positive predictive value of only 6% (in other words, it picks up almost all babies with the condition at the expense of a high false positive rate), [11] and rightly so. It is far more important to pick up every single baby with this treatable condition who would otherwise develop severe mental handicap than to save hundreds of parents the relatively minor stress of a repeat blood test on their baby.

Question 8: were confidence intervals given for sensitivity, specificity and other features of the test?

As Section 5.5 explained, a confidence interval, which can be calculated for virtually every numerical aspect of a set of results, expresses the possible range of results within which the true value will lie. Go back to the jury example in Section 7.1. If they had found just one more murderer not guilty, the sensitivity of their verdict would have gone down from 67% to 33%, and the positive predictive value of the verdict from 33% to 20%. This enormous (and quite unacceptable) sensitivity to a single case decision is, of course, because we only validated the jury's performance on 10 cases. The confidence intervals for the features of this jury are so wide that my computer programme refuses to calculate them! Remember, the larger the sample size, the narrower the confidence interval, so it is particularly important to look for confidence intervals if the paper you are reading reports a study on a relatively small sample. If you would like the formula for calculating confidence intervals for diagnostic test features, see the excellent textbook *Statistics with confidence.*[12]

Question 9: has a sensible 'normal range' been derived from these results?

If the test gives non-dichotomous (continuous) results – that is, if it gives a numerical value rather than a yes/no result – someone will have to say at what value the test result will count as abnormal. Many of us have been there with our own blood pressure reading. We want to know if our result is 'okay' or not, but the doctor insists on giving us a value such as '142/92'. If 140/90 were chosen as the cut-off for high blood pressure, we would be placed in the 'abnormal' category, even though our risk of problems from our blood pressure is very little different from that of a person with a blood pressure of 138/88. Quite sensibly, many practising doctors advise their patients, 'Your blood pressure isn't quite right, but it doesn't fall into the danger zone. Come back in three months for another check'. Nevertheless, the doctor must at some stage make the decision that *this* blood pressure needs treating with tablets but *this* one does not.

Defining relative and absolute danger zones for a continuous physiological or pathological variable is a complex science which should take into account the actual likelihood of the adverse outcome which the proposed treatment aims to prevent. This process is made considerably more objective by the use of likelihood ratios (see Section 7.4). For an entertaining discussion on the different possible meanings of the word 'normal' in diagnostic investigations, see Sackett and colleagues' textbook, p. 59. [6]

Question 10: has this test been placed in the context of other potential tests in the diagnostic sequence for the condition?

In general, we treat high blood pressure simply on the basis of the blood pressure reading alone (although we tend to rely on a series of readings rather than a single value). Compare this with the sequence we use to diagnose stenosis ('hardening') of the coronary arteries. First, we select patients with a typical history of effort angina (chest pain on exercise). Next, we usually do a resting ECG, an exercise ECG, and, in some cases, a radionuclide scan of the heart to look for areas short of oxygen. Most patients only come to a coronary angiogram (the definitive investigation for coronary artery stenosis) *after* they have produced an abnormal result on these preliminary tests.

If you took 100 people off the street and sent them straight for a coronary angiogram, the test might display very different positive and negative predictive values (and even different sensitivity and specificity) than it did in the sicker population on which it was originally validated. This means that the various aspects of validity of the coronary angiogram as a diagnostic test are virtually meaningless unless these figures are expressed in terms of what they contribute to the overall diagnostic work-up.

7.4 A note on likelihood ratios

Question 9 above described the problem of defining a normal range for a continuous variable. In such circumstances, it can be preferable to express the test result not as 'normal' or 'abnormal', but in terms of the actual chances of a patient having the target disorder if the test result reaches a particular level. Take, for example, the use of the prostate-specific antigen (PSA) test to screen for prostate cancer. Most men will have some detectable PSA in their blood (say, 0.5 ng/ml), and most of those with advanced prostate cancer will have very high levels of PSA (above about 20 ng/ml). But a PSA level of, say, 7.4 ng/ml may be found either in a perfectly normal man or in someone with early cancer. There simply is not a clean cut-off between normal and abnormal. [13]

We can, however, use the results of a validation study of the PSA test against a gold standard for prostate cancer (say a biopsy) to draw up a whole series of 2 × 2 tables. Each table would use a different definition of an abnormal PSA result to classify patients as 'normal' or 'abnormal'. From these tables, we could generate different likelihood ratios associated with a PSA level above each different cut-off point. Then, when faced with a PSA result in the 'grey zone', we would at least be able to say, 'this test has not proved that the patient has prostate cancer, but it has increased (or decreased) the odds of that diagnosis by a factor of *x*'. (In fact, as I mentioned in Section 6.3, the PSA test is not a terribly good discriminator between the presence and absence of cancer, whatever cut-off value is used – in other words, there is no value for PSA that gives a particularly high likelihood ratio in cancer detection.)

Although the likelihood ratio is one of the more complicated aspects of a diagnostic test to calculate, it has enormous practical value, and it is becoming the preferred way of expressing and comparing the usefulness of different tests. As Sackett and colleagues explain at great length in their textbook, [6] the likelihood ratio can be used directly in ruling a particular diagnosis in or out. For example, if a person enters my consulting room with no symptoms

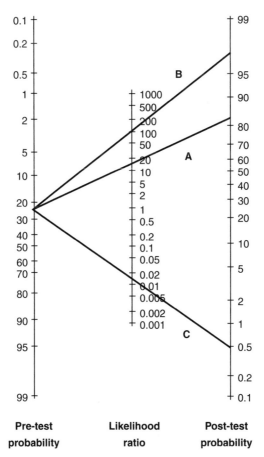

Figure 7.4 Likelihood ratio nomogram: using likelihood ratios to calculate the post-test probability of someone being a smoker.

at all, I know that they have a 5% chance of having iron-deficiency anaemia, since I know that one person in 20 in the population has this condition (in the language of diagnostic tests, this means that the pre-test probability of anaemia, equivalent to the prevalence of the condition, is 0.05). [14]

Now, if I do a diagnostic test for anaemia, the serum ferritin level, the result will usually make the diagnosis of anaemia either more or less likely. A moderately reduced serum ferritin level (between 18 and 45 μg/l) has a likelihood ratio of 3, so the chances of a patient with this result having iron deficiency anaemia is generally calculated as 0.05 × 3, or 0.15 (15%). This value is known as the post-test probability of the serum ferritin test.

(Strictly speaking, likelihood ratios should be used on odds rather than on probabilities, but the simpler method shown here gives a good approximation when the pre-test probability is low. In this example, a pre-test probability of 5% is equal to a pre-test odds of 0.05/0.95 or 0.053; a positive test with a likelihood ratio of 3 gives a post-test odds of 0.158, which is equal to a post-test probability of 14%.)[14]

Figure 7.4 shows a nomogram, adapted by Sackett and colleagues from an original paper by Fagan, [15] for working out post-test probabilities when the pre-test probability (prevalence) and likelihood ratio for the test are known. The lines A, B and C, drawn from a pre-test probability of 25% (the prevalence of smoking amongst British adults) are, respectively, the trajectories through likelihood ratios of 15, 100 and 0.015 – three different tests for detecting whether someone is a smoker or not. [16] Actually, test C detects whether the person is a *non-smoker*, since a positive result in this test leads to a post-test probability of only 0.5%.

In summary, as I said at the beginning of this chapter, you can get a long way with diagnostic tests without referring to likelihood ratios. I avoided them myself for years. But if you put aside an afternoon to get to grips with this aspect of clinical epidemiology, I predict that your time will have been well spent.

References

1 Kuzuya T, Nakagawa S, Satoh J, Kanazawa Y, Iwamoto Y, Kobayashi M *et al.* Report of the Committee on the classification and diagnostic criteria of diabetes mellitus. *Diabetes Res Clin Pract* 2002;**55**:65–85.

2 Andersson DK, Lundblad E, Svardsudd K. A model for early diagnosis of type 2 diabetes mellitus in primary health care. *Diabet Med* 1993;**10**:167–73.

3 Friderichsen B, Maunsbach M. Glycosuric tests should not be employed in population screenings for NIDDM. *J Public Health Med* 1997;**19**:55–60.

4 Jaeschke R, Guyatt GH, Sackett DL. Users' guides to the medical literature. III. How to use an article about a diagnostic test. B. What are the results and will they help me in caring for my patients? Evidence-Based Medicine Working Group. *JAMA* 1994;**271**:703–7.

5 Jaeschke R, Guyatt GH, Sackett DL. Users' guides to the medical literature. III. How to use an article about a diagnostic test. A. Are the results of the study valid? Evidence-Based Medicine Working Group. *JAMA* 1994;**271**:389–91.

6 Sackett DL, Haynes RB, Guyatt GH, Tugwell P. *Clinical epidemiology. A basic science for clinical medicine.* Boston: Little Brown & Company, 1991.

7 Reid MC, Lachs MS, Feinstein AR. Use of methodological standards in diagnostic test research. Getting better but still not good. *JAMA* 1995;**274**:645–51.

8 Mant D. Testing a test: three critical steps. In: Jones R, Kinmonth A-L, eds. *Critical reading for primary care.* Oxford: Oxford University Press, 1995.

9 Whiting P, Rutjes AW, Dinnes J, Reitsma J, Bossuyt PM, Kleijnen J. Development and validation of methods for assessing the quality of diagnostic accuracy studies. *Health Technol Assess* 2004;**8**(iii):1–234.

10 Bush B, Shaw S, Cleary P, Delbanco TL, Aronson MD. Screening for alcohol abuse using the CAGE questionnaire. *Am J Med* 1987;**82**:231–5.

11 Verkerk PH, Derksen-Lubsen G, Vulsma T, Loeber JG, de Vijlder JJ, Verbrugge HP. [Evaluation of a decade of neonatal screening for congenital hypothyroidism in The Netherlands]. *Ned Tijdschr Geneeskd* 1993;**137**:2199–205.

12 Gardner M, Altman DG, Bryant T, Machin D. *Statistics with confidence: confidence intervals and statistical guidelines.* London: BMJ Books, 2000.

13 Catalona WJ, Hudson MA, Scardino PT, Richie JP, Ahmann FR, Flanigan RC *et al.* Selection of optimal prostate specific antigen cutoffs for early detection of prostate cancer: receiver operating characteristic curves. *J Urol* 1994;**152**:2037–42.

14 Guyatt GH, Patterson C, Ali M, Singer J, Levine M, Turpie I *et al.* Diagnosis of iron-deficiency anemia in the elderly. *Am J Med* 1990;**88**:205–9.

15 Fagan TJ. Letter: nomogram for Bayes theorem. *N Engl J Med* 1975;**293**:257.

16 Anonymous. How good is that test – using the result. *Bandolier* 1996;**3**:6–8.

Chapter 8 **Papers that summarise other papers (systematic reviews and meta-analyses)**

8.1 When is a review systematic?

Remember the essays you used to write when you first started college? You would mooch round the library, browsing through the indexes of books and journals. When you came across a paragraph that looked relevant you copied it out, and if anything you found did not fit in with the theory you were proposing, you left it out. This, more or less, constitutes the *journalistic* review – an overview of primary studies which have not been identified or analysed in a systematic (i.e. standardised and objective) way. Journalists get paid according to how much they write rather than how much they read or how critically they process it, which explains why most of the 'new scientific breakthroughs' you read in your newspaper today will probably be discredited before the month is out. A common variant of the journalistic review is the invited review, written when an editor asks one of his or her friends to pen a piece, and summed up by this fabulous title: 'The invited review? Or, my field, from my standpoint, written by me using only my data and my ideas, and citing only my publications'![1]

In contrast, a *systematic review* is an overview of primary studies which
- contains a statement of objectives, materials and methods;
- has been conducted according to explicit, transparent and reproducible method (see Figure 8.1)

The most enduring and useful systematic reviews, notably those undertaken by the Cochrane Collaboration (see Section 2.10) are regularly updated to incorporate new evidence.

Many, if not most, medical review articles are still written in journalistic form. Professor Paul Knipschild, in the first edition of Iain Chalmers's and Doug Altman's excellent book, *Systematic reviews*,[2] describes how Nobel Prize winning biochemist Linus Pauling used selective quotes from the medical literature to 'prove' his theory that vitamin C helps you live longer and feel better.[3] When Knipschild and his colleagues searched the literature

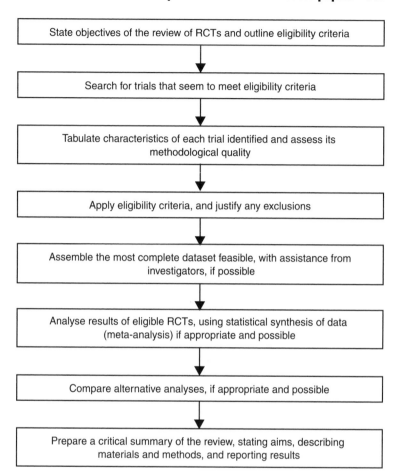

Figure 8.1 Method for a systematic review.

systematically for evidence for and against this hypothesis, they found that although one or two trials did strongly suggest that vitamin C could prevent the onset of the common cold, there were far more studies that did not show any beneficial effect.

Linus Pauling probably did not deliberately intend to deceive his readers, but since his enthusiasm for his espoused cause outweighed his scientific objectivity, he was unaware of the *selection bias* influencing his choice of papers. Much work has been done, most notably by Professor Cindy Mulrow and her team of the University of Texas Health Science Center, USA, which confirms the sneaky feeling that were you or I to attempt what Pauling

> **Box 8.1** Advantages of systematic reviews (see reference 2)
>
> 1　Explicit methods *limit bias* in identifying and rejecting studies.
> 2　Conclusions are hence more *reliable* and *accurate*.
> 3　Large amounts of *information* can be assimilated quickly by health care providers, researchers and policy makers.
> 4　Delay between research discoveries and *implementation* of effective diagnostic and therapeutic strategies is reduced (see Chapter 12).
> 5　Results of different studies can be formally compared to establish *generalisability* of findings and *consistency* (lack of heterogeneity) of results (see Section 8.4).
> 6　Reasons for *heterogeneity* (inconsistency in results across studies) can be identified and new hypotheses generated about particular subgroups (see Section 8.4).
> 7　Quantitative systematic reviews (meta-analyses) increase the *precision* of the overall result (see Sections 4.6 and 8.3).

did – that is, hunt through the medical literature for 'evidence' to support our pet theory – we would make an equally idiosyncratic and unscientific job of it.[4,5] Mulrow, along with Iain Chalmers at the UK Cochrane Centre and Peter Gotzsche and Andy Oxman of the Nordic Cochrane Centre (see Section 2.10), deserves much of the credit for persuading the rest of the medical community that flawed secondary research, exemplified by the journalistic review, is as scientifically dangerous as flawed primary research. Some advantages of the systematic review are given in Box 8.1.

Experts, who have been steeped in a subject for years and know what the answer 'ought' to be, were once shown to be significantly less able to produce an objective review of the literature in their subject than non-experts.[6] This would have been of little consequence if experts' opinion could be relied upon to be congruent with the results of independent systematic reviews, but at the time they most certainly couldn't.[7] These condemning studies are still widely quoted by people who would replace all subject experts (such as cardiologists) with search-and-appraisal experts (people who specialise in finding and criticising papers on any subject). But no one in more recent years has replicated the findings – in other words, perhaps we should credit today's experts with more of a tendency to base their recommendations on a thorough assessment of the evidence! As a general rule, however, if you are going to pay someone to seek out the best objective evidence of the benefits of anticoagulants in atrial fibrillation, you should ask someone who is an expert in systematic reviews to work alongside an expert in atrial fibrillation.

To be fair to Linus Pauling, he did mention a number of trials the results of which seriously challenged his theory that vitamin C prevents the common cold.[3] But he described all such trials as 'methodologically flawed'. As Knipschild reminds us, so were many of the trials which Pauling *did* include in his analysis, but because their results were consistent with the theory, Pauling was, perhaps subconsciously, less critical of weaknesses in their design.

I mention this example to illustrate the point that, when undertaking a systematic review, not only must the search for relevant articles be thorough and objective, but the criteria used to reject articles as 'flawed' must also be explicit and independent of the results of those trials. In other words, you don't trash a trial because all other trials in this area showed something different (see Section 8.4); you trash it because, *whatever the results showed*, the trial's objectives or methods did not meet your inclusion criteria or quality standard (see Section 3.1).

8.2 Evaluating systematic reviews

One of the major developments in EBM since I wrote the first edition of this book in 1995 has been the agreement on a standard, structured format for writing up and presenting systematic reviews.[8] This QUORUM format (equivalent to the CONSORT format for reporting randomised controlled trials discussed in Section 3.3) makes them a whole lot easier to find your way around. Here are some questions to ask about any systematic review of quantitative evidence.

Question 1: can you find an important clinical question which the review addressed?

Look back to Chapter 3 in which I explained the importance of defining the question when reading a paper about a clinical trial or other form of primary research. I called this 'getting your bearings' since one sure way to be confused about a paper is to fail to ascertain what it is about. The definition of a specific answerable question is, if anything, even more important (and even more frequently omitted!) when preparing an overview of primary studies. If you have ever tried to pull together the findings of a dozen or more clinical papers into an essay, editorial or summary notes for an examination, you will know that it is all too easy to meander into aspects of the subject which you never intended to cover.

The question addressed by a systematic review needs to be defined very precisely, since the reviewer must make a dichotomous (yes/no) decision as to whether each potentially relevant paper will be included or, alternatively, rejected as 'irrelevant'. The question, 'do anticoagulants prevent strokes in patients with atrial fibrillation?' sounds pretty specific until you start looking through the list of possible studies to include. Does 'atrial fibrillation' include both rheumatic and non-rheumatic forms (which are known to be associated with very different risks of stroke), and does it include intermittent atrial fibrillation (my grandfather, e.g. used to go into this arrhythmia for a few hours whenever he drank coffee and would have counted as a 'grey case' in any trial)?

Does 'stroke' include both ischaemic stroke (caused by a *blocked* blood vessel in the brain) and haemorrhagic stroke (caused by a *burst* blood vessel)? And, talking of burst blood vessels, shouldn't we be weighing the side effects of anticoagulants against their possible benefits? Should true anticoagulants such as heparin and warfarin be compared with placebo, or should they be compared with other drugs that reduce the clotting tendency of the blood, such as aspirin and related products? Finally, should the review cover trials on patients who have already had a previous stroke or transient ischaemic attack (a mild stroke that gets better within 24 h), or should it be limited to trials on patients without these major risk factors for a further stroke? The 'simple' question posed earlier is becoming unanswerable, and we must refine it as follows:

> To assess the effectiveness and safety of warfarin-type anticoagulant therapy in secondary prevention (i.e. following a previous stroke or transient ischaemic attack) in patients with non-rheumatic atrial fibrillation: comparison with placebo.[9]

Question 2: was a thorough search done of the appropriate database(s) and were other potentially important sources explored?

As Figure 8.1 illustrates, one of the benefits of a systematic review is that, unlike a narrative or journalistic review, the author is required to tell you where the information in it came from and how it was processed. As I explained in Chapter 2, searching the Medline database for relevant articles is a very sophisticated science, and even the best Medline search will miss important papers. The reviewer who seeks a comprehensive set of primary studies must approach the other databases listed in Section 2.10 – and sometimes many more (e.g. in a recent systematic review of the diffusion of innovations in health service organisations, my colleagues and I searched a total of 15 databases, 9 of which I'd never even heard of when I started the study[10]).

In the search for trials to include in a review, the scrupulous avoidance of linguistic imperialism is a scientific as well as a political imperative. As much weight must be given, for example, to the expressions 'Eine Placebo-kontrolierte Doppel-blindstudie' and 'une étude randomisée a double insu face au placebo' as to 'a double-blind, randomised controlled trial',[3] although Moher has shown that omission of other-language studies does not tend to bias the result (it's just bad science).[11] Furthermore, particularly where a statistical synthesis of results (meta-analysis) is contemplated, it may be necessary to write and ask the authors of the primary studies for data that were not originally included in the published review (see Section 8.3).

Even when all this has been done, the systematic reviewer's search for material has hardly begun. As Paul Knipschild and his colleagues showed when they searched for trials on vitamin C and cold prevention, their electronic databases only gave them 22 of their final total of 61 trials.[2] Another 39 trials were uncovered by hand-searching the manual Index Medicus database (14 trials not identified previously), and searching the references of the trials identified in Medline (15 more trials), the references of the references (9 further trials), and the references of the references of the references (1 additional trial not identified by any of the previous searches).

Do not be too hard on a reviewer, however, if he or she has not followed this counsel of perfection to the letter. After all, Knipschild and his team found that only one of the trials not identified in Medline met stringent criteria for methodological quality and ultimately contributed to their systematic review of vitamin C in cold prevention.[2] The use of more laborious search methods (such as pursuing the references of references, writing to all the known experts in the field, and hunting out 'grey literature') (see Box 8.2) may be of greater relative importance when looking at trials outside the medical mainstream. For example, in health service management, my own team recently showed that only around a quarter of relevant, high quality papers were turned up by electronic searching.[12]

Question 3: was methodological quality assessed and the trials weighted accordingly?

Chapters 3 and 4 and Appendix 1 of this book provide some checklists for assessing whether a paper should be rejected outright on methodological grounds. But given that only around 1% of clinical trials are said to be beyond criticism methodologically, the practical question is how to ensure that a 'small but perfectly formed' study is given the weight it deserves in relation to a larger study whose methods are adequate but more open to criticism.

Box 8.2 Checklist of data sources for a systematic review

• Medline database
• Cochrane controlled clinical trials register (see Section 2.10)
• Other medical and paramedical databases (see Section 2.10)
• Foreign language literature
• 'Grey literature' (theses, internal reports, non-peer reviewed journals, pharmaceutical industry files)
• References (and references of references, etc.) listed in primary sources
• Other unpublished sources known to experts in the field (seek by personal communication)
• Raw data from published trials (seek by personal communication).

Methodological shortcomings which invalidate the results of trials are often generic (i.e. they are independent of the subject matter of the study; see Appendix 1), but there may also be particular methodological features which distinguish between good, medium and poor quality in a particular field. Hence, one of the tasks of a systematic reviewer is to draw up a list of criteria, including both generic and particular aspects of quality, against which to judge each trial. In theory, a composite numerical score could be calculated which would reflect 'overall methodological quality'. In reality, however, care should be taken in developing such scores since there is no gold standard for the 'true' methodological quality of a trial[13] and such composite scores may prove neither valid nor reliable in practice.[14,15] If you're interested in reading more about the science of developing and applying quality criteria to studies as part of a systematic review, see the references listed at the end of this chapter.[14–17]

Question 4: how sensitive are the results to the way the review has been done?

If you don't understand what this question means, look up the tongue-in-cheek paper by Carl Counsell and colleagues in the Christmas 1994 issue of the *British Medical Journal*, which 'proved' an entirely spurious relationship between the result of shaking a dice and the outcome of an acute stroke.[18] The authors report a series of artificial dice-rolling experiments in which red, white and green dice respectively represented different therapies for acute stroke.

Overall, the 'trials' showed no significant benefit from the three therapies. However, the simulation of a number of perfectly plausible events in the process of meta-analysis – such as the exclusion of several of the 'negative' trials through publication bias (see Section 3.3), a subgroup analysis which excluded data on red dice therapy (since, on looking back at the results, red dice appeared to be harmful) and other, essentially arbitrary, exclusions on the grounds of 'methodological quality' – led to an apparently highly significant benefit of 'dice therapy' in acute stroke.

You cannot, of course, cure anyone of a stroke by rolling a dice, but if these simulated results pertained to a genuine medical controversy (such as which groups of postmenopausal women should take hormone replacement therapy or whether breech babies should routinely be delivered by Caesarean section), how would you spot these subtle biases? The answer is you need to work through the what-ifs. What if the authors of the systematic review had changed the inclusion criteria? What if they had excluded unpublished studies? What if their 'quality weightings' had been assigned differently? What if trials of lower methodological quality had been included (or excluded)? What if all the unaccounted-for patients in a trial were assumed to have died (or been cured)?

An exploration of what-ifs is known as a *sensitivity analysis*. If you find that fiddling with the data like this in various ways makes little or no difference to the review's overall results, you can assume that the review's conclusions are relatively robust. If, however, the key findings disappear when any of the what-ifs change, the conclusions should be expressed far more cautiously and you should hesitate before changing your practice in the light of them.

Question 5: have the numerical results been interpreted with common sense and due regard to the broader aspects of the problem?

As Section 8.3 shows, it is easy to be 'phased' by the figures and graphs in a systematic review. But any numerical result, however precise, accurate, 'significant', or otherwise incontrovertible, must be placed in the context of the painfully simple and (often) frustratingly general question which the review addressed. The clinician must decide how (if at all) this numerical result, *whether significant or not*, should influence the care of an individual patient.

A particularly important feature to consider when undertaking or appraising a systematic review is the external validity of included trials (see Box 8.3). A trial may be of high methodological quality and have a precise and numerically impressive result, but it may, for example, have been conducted on participants under the age of 60, and hence may not be valid for people over 75. The inclusion in systematic reviews of irrelevant studies is guaranteed

> **Box 8.3** Assigning weight to trials in a systematic review
>
> Each trial should be evaluated in terms of its
> 1 *methodological quality* – that is, extent to which the design and conduct are likely to have prevented systematic errors (bias) (see Section 4.4);
> 2 *precision* – that is, a measure of the likelihood of random errors (usually depicted as the width of the confidence interval around the result);
> 3 *external validity* – that is, the extent to which the results are generalisable or applicable to a particular target population.
> (Additional aspects of 'quality', such as scientific importance, clinical importance and literary quality, are rightly given great weight by peer reviewers and journal editors, but are less relevant to the systematic reviewer once the question to be addressed has been defined.)

to lead to absurdities and reduce the credibility of secondary research, as Professor Sir John Grimley Evans has argued (see quote in Section 9.1).[19]

8.3 Meta-analysis for the non-statistician

If I had to pick one word which exemplifies the fear and loathing felt by so many students, clinicians and consumers towards evidence-based medicine, it would be 'meta-analysis'. The meta-analysis, defined as *a statistical synthesis of the numerical results of several trials which all addressed the same question*, is the statisticians' chance to pull a double whammy on you. First, they phase you with all the statistical tests in the individual papers, and then they use a whole new battery of tests to produce a new set of odds ratios, confidence intervals and values for significance.

As I confessed in Chapter 5, I too tend to go into a panic mode at the sight of ratios, square root signs and half-forgotten Greek letters. But before you consign meta-analysis to the set of newfangled techniques which you will never understand, remember two things. First, the meta-analyst may wear an anorak but he or she is *on your side*. A good meta-analysis is often easier for the non-statistician to understand than the stack of primary research papers from which it was derived, for reasons I am about to explain. Second, the underlying statistical techniques used for meta-analysis are exactly the same as the ones for any other data analysis – it's just that some of the numbers are bigger.

The first task of the meta-analyst, after following the preliminary steps for systematic review in Figure 8.1, is to decide which out of all the various outcome measures chosen by the authors of the primary studies is the best one (or ones) to use in the overall synthesis. In trials of a particular chemotherapy regimen for breast cancer, for example, some authors will have published cumulative mortality figures (i.e. the total number of people who have died to date) at cutoff points of 3 and 12 months, whereas other trials will have published 6-month, 12-month and 5-year cumulative mortality. The meta-analyst might decide to concentrate on 12-month mortality because this result can be easily extracted from all the papers. He or she may, however, decide that 3-month mortality is a clinically important end point and would need to write to the authors of the remaining trials asking for the raw data from which to calculate these figures.

In addition to crunching the numbers, part of the meta-analyst's job description is to tabulate relevant information on the inclusion criteria, sample size, baseline patient characteristics, withdrawal ('drop-out') rate and results of primary and secondary end points of all the studies included. If this task has been done properly, you will be able to compare both the methods and the results of two trials whose authors wrote up their research in different ways. Although such tables are often visually daunting, they save you from having to plough through the methods sections of each paper and compare one author's tabulated results with another author's pie chart or histogram.

These days the results of meta-analyses tend to be presented in a fairly standard form. This is partly because meta-analysts often use computer software to do the calculations for them (see the latest edition of the *Cochrane Reviewers' handbook* for an up-to-date menu of options[14]), and most such software packages include a standard graphics tool which presents results as illustrated in Figure 8.2. I have reproduced in the format of one commonly used software package (with the authors' permission) this pictorial representation (colloquially known as a 'forest plot' or 'blobbogram') of the pooled odds ratios of eight randomised controlled trials which each compared coronary artery bypass graft (CABG) with percutaneous coronary angioplasty (PTCA) in the treatment of severe angina.[21] The primary (main) outcome in this meta-analysis was death or heart attack within 1 year.

The eight trials, each represented by its acronym (e.g. 'CABRI'), are listed one below the other on the left-hand side of the figure. The horizontal line corresponding to each trial shows the relative risk (RR) of death or heart attack at 1 year in patients randomised to PTCA compared with patients randomised to CABG. The 'blob' in the middle of each line is the point estimate of the difference between the groups (the best single estimate of the benefit in lives saved by offering CABG rather than PTCA), and the width of the line represents the 95% confidence interval of this estimate (see Section 5.5b). The black line down the middle of the picture is known as the 'line of no effect', and in this case is associated with a relative risk of 1.0.

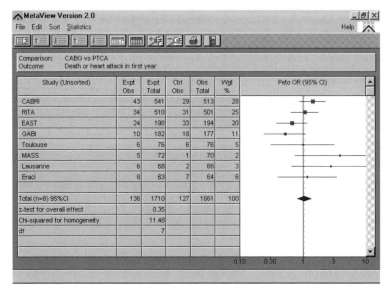

Figure 8.2 Pooled odds ratios of eight RCTs of coronary artery bypass graft against percutaneous coronary angiography, shown in MetaView format (see reference 20).

In other words, if the horizontal line for any trial does not cross the line of no effect, there is a 95% chance that there is a 'real' difference between the groups.

As Sections 4.6 and 5.5 argued, if the confidence interval of the result (the horizontal line) *does* cross the line of no effect (i.e. the vertical line), this can mean *either* that there is no significant difference between the treatments *and/or* that the sample size was too small to allow us to be confident where the true result lies. The various individual studies give point estimates of the relative risk of PTCA compared with CABG (of between about 0.5 and 5.0), and the confidence intervals of some studies are so wide that they don't even fit on the graph.

Now, here comes the fun of meta-analysis. Look at the tiny diamond below all the horizontal lines. This represents the *pooled* data from all eight trials (overall relative risk PTCA : CABG = 1.08), with a new, much narrower, confidence interval of this relative risk (0.79 −1.50). Since the diamond firmly overlaps the line of no effect, we can say that there is probably little to choose between the two treatments in terms of the primary end point (death or heart attack in the first year). Now, in this example, every single one of the eight trials also suggested a non-significant effect, but in none of them was the sample size large enough for us to be *confident* in that negative result.

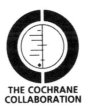

**THE COCHRANE
COLLABORATION**

Figure 8.3 Cochrane Collaboration logo.

Note, however, that this neat little diamond does *not* mean that you might as well offer a PTCA rather than a CABG to every patient with angina. It has a much more limited meaning – that the *average* patient in the trials presented in this meta-analysis is equally likely to have met the primary outcome (death or heart attack within a year) whichever of these two treatments they were randomised to receive. If you read the paper by Pocock and colleagues,[21] you would find important differences in the groups in terms of prevalence of angina and requirement for further operative intervention after the initial procedure. The choice of treatment should also, of course, take into account how the patient feels about undergoing major heart surgery (CABG) as opposed to the relatively minor procedure of PTCA.

In many meta-analyses, 'non-significant' trials (i.e. ones which, on their own, did not demonstrate a significant difference between treatment and control groups) contribute to a pooled result which *is* statistically significant. The most famous example of this, which the Cochrane Collaboration adopted as its logo (Figure 8.3), is the meta-analysis of seven trials of the effect of giving steroids to mothers who were expected to give birth prematurely.[22] Only two of the seven trials showed a statistically significant benefit (in terms of survival of the infant), but the improvement in precision (i.e. the narrowing of confidence intervals) in the pooled results, shown by the narrower width of the diamond compared with the individual lines, demonstrates the strength of the evidence in favour of this intervention. This meta-analysis showed that infants of steroid-treated mothers were 30–50% less likely to die than infants of control mothers. This example is discussed further in Section 12.1 in relation to changing clinicians' behaviour.

You may have worked out by now that anyone who is thinking about doing a clinical trial of an intervention should first do a meta-analysis of all the previous trials on that same intervention. In practice, researchers rarely do this. Dean Fergusson and colleagues of the Ottawa Health Research Institute recently published a cumulative meta-analysis of all randomised controlled trials done on the drug aprotinin in perioperative bleeding during cardiac surgery.[20] They lined up the trials in the order they had been published, and worked out what a meta-analysis of 'all trials done so far' would have shown (had it been done at the time). The resulting *cumulative meta-analysis* had shocking news for the research communities. The beneficial effect of aprotinin reached statistical significance after only 12 trials – that is, back in 1992. But because nobody did a meta-analysis at the time, a further 52 clinical trials were undertaken (and more are ongoing). All these trials were scientifically unnecessary and unethical (since half the patients were denied a drug that had been proven to improve outcome). Figure 8.4 illustrates this waste of effort.

If you have followed the arguments on meta-analysis of published trial results this far, you might like to read up on the more sophisticated technique of meta-analysis of individual patient data, which provides a more accurate and precise figure for the point estimate of effect.[24] You might also like to seek out the excellent review series on meta-analysis published in the *British Medical Journal* a few years ago,[23,25] and subsequent methodological articles by the same group of authors.[30,31]

8.4 Explaining heterogeneity

In everyday language, 'homogeneous' means 'of uniform composition', and 'heterogeneous' means 'many different ingredients'. In the language of meta-analysis, homogeneity means that the results of each individual trial are compatible with the results of any of the others. Homogeneity can be estimated at a glance once the trial results have been presented in the format illustrated in Figures 8.2 and 8.5. In Figure 8.2, the lower confidence interval of every trial is below the upper confidence interval of all the others (i.e. the horizontal lines all overlap to some extent). Statistically speaking, the trials are homogeneous. Conversely, in Figure 8.5, there are some trials whose lower confidence interval is above the upper confidence interval of one or more other trials (i.e. some lines do not overlap at all). These trials may be said to be heterogeneous.

You may have spotted by now (particularly if you have already read Section 5.5b on confidence intervals) that pronouncing a set of trials heterogeneous on the basis of whether their confidence intervals overlap is somewhat arbitrary, since the confidence interval itself is arbitrary (it can be set at 90%, 95%, 99% or indeed any other value). The definitive test involves a slightly more sophisticated statistical manoeuvre than holding a ruler up against the blobbogram. The one most commonly used is a variant of the Chi-square (χ^2) test (see Table 5.1 in Chapter 5), since the question addressed is, 'is there greater variation between the results of the trials than is compatible with the play of chance'?

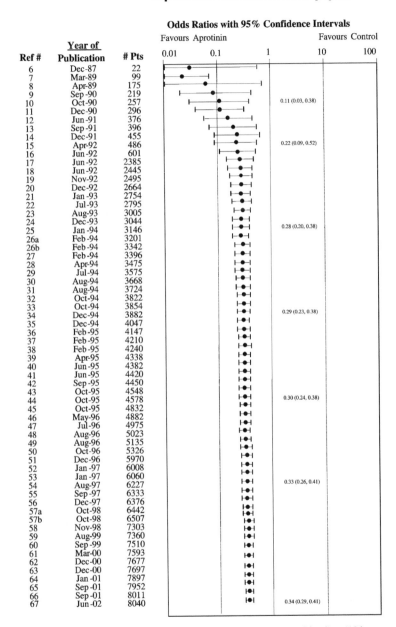

Figure 8.4 Cumulative meta-analysis of aprotinin in perioperative bleeding. With permission from Fergusson D *et al*. Randomised controlled trials of aprotinin in cardiac surgery: could clinical equipoise have stopped the bleeding? *Clinical Trials* 2005;**2**:218–32.

The χ^2 statistic for heterogeneity is explained in more detail by Simon Thompson,[32] who offers the following useful rule of thumb: a χ^2 statistic has, on average, a value equal to its degrees of freedom (in this case, the number of trials in the meta-analysis minus one), so a χ^2 of 7.0 for a set of eight trials would provide no evidence of statistical heterogeneity. (In fact, it would not prove that the trials were homogeneous either, particularly since the χ^2 test has low power [see Section 4.6] to detect small but important levels of heterogeneity.)

A χ^2 value much greater than the number of trials in a meta-analysis tells us that the trials which contributed to the analysis are different in some important way from one another. There may, for example, be known differences in method (e.g. authors may have used different questionnaires to assess the symptoms of depression) or known clinical differences in the trial participants (e.g. one centre might have been a tertiary referral hospital to which all the sickest patients were referred). There may, however, be unknown or unrecorded differences between the trials which the meta-analyst can only speculate upon until he or she has extracted further details from the trials' authors. Remember: demonstrating statistical heterogeneity is a mathematical exercise and is the job of the statistician, but explaining this heterogeneity (i.e. looking for, and accounting for, *clinical* heterogeneity) is an interpretive exercise and requires imagination, common sense, and hands-on clinical or research experience.

Figure 8.5, which is reproduced with permission from Simon Thompson's chapter on the subject,[32] shows the results of 10 trials of cholesterol-lowering strategies. The results are expressed as the percentage reduction in heart disease risk associated with each 0.6 mmol/l reduction in serum cholesterol level. The horizontal lines represent the 95% confidence intervals of each result, and it is clear, even without being told the χ^2 statistic of 127, that the trials are highly heterogeneous.

To simply 'average out' the results of the trials in Figure 8.5 would be very misleading. The meta-analyst must return to his or her primary sources and ask, 'in what way was trial A different from trial B, and what do trials C, D and H have in common which makes their results cluster at one extreme of the figure'? In this example, a correction for the age of the trial subjects reduced χ^2 from 127 to 45. In other words, most of the 'incompatibility' in the results of these trials can be explained by the fact that embarking on a strategy (such as a special diet) which successfully reduces your cholesterol level will be substantially more likely to prevent a heart attack if you are 45 than if you are 85.

This, essentially, is the essence of the grievance of Professor Hans Eysenck who has constructed a vigorous and entertaining critique of the science of

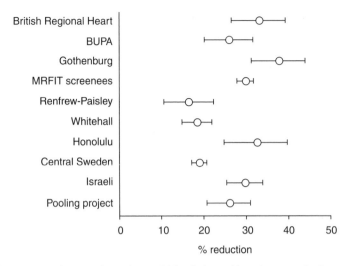

Figure 8.5 Reduction in heart disease risk by cholesterol lowering strategies (see reference 23).

meta-analysis.[33] In a world of lumpers and splitters, Eysenck is a splitter, and it offends his sense of the qualitative and the particular (see Chapter 11) to combine the results of studies which were done on different populations in different places at different times and for different reasons.

Eysenck's reservations about meta-analysis are borne out in the infamously discredited meta-analysis which demonstrated (wrongly) that there was significant benefit to be had from giving intravenous magnesium to heart attack victims. A subsequent megatrial involving 58,000 patients (ISIS-4) failed to find any benefit whatsoever, and the meta-analysts' misleading conclusions were subsequently explained in terms of publication bias, methodological weaknesses in the smaller trials and clinical heterogeneity.[34,35] (Incidentally, for more debate on the pros and cons of meta-analysis versus megatrials, see LeLorier and colleagues' *Lancet* article.[36])

Eysenck's mathematical naiveté is embarrassing ('if a medical treatment has an effect so recondite and obscure as to require a meta-analysis to establish it, I would not be happy to have it used on me'), which is perhaps why the editors of the second edition of the *Systematic reviews* book dropped his chapter from their collection. But I have a great deal of sympathy for the principle of his argument. As one who tends to side with the splitters, I would put Eysenck's misgivings about meta-analysis high on the list of required reading for the aspiring systematic reviewer. Indeed, I once threw my own hat into the ring when Simon Griffin published a meta-analysis of primary studies into the management of diabetes by primary health care teams.[37] Although I have a high regard for Simon as a scientist, I felt strongly that he had not been justified in performing a mathematical summation of what I believed were very different studies all addressing slightly different questions. As I said in my commentary on his article, 'four apples and five oranges makes four apples and five oranges, not nine appleoranges'.[38] But Simon numbers himself among the lumpers, and there are plenty of people cleverer than me who have argued that he was entirely correct to analyse his data as he did. Fortunately, the two of us have agreed to differ – and on a personal level we remain friends.

8.5 New approaches to systematic review

This chapter has addressed the most commonly used approach to systematic review – synthesising trials of therapy. If you're comfortable with that, you might like to start exploring the literature on systematic review of observational (cohort) studies,[39–41] diagnostic and screening tests,[42,43] alternative therapies,[44] educational interventions,[45] economic evaluation[46,47] and the emerging science of systematic review of qualitative research (and mixed qualitative and quantitative studies), which I discuss in more detail in Chapter 11.[48,49] For my own part, I've been working with colleagues to develop new approaches to systematic review that highlight and explore (rather than attempt to 'average out') the fundamental differences between primary studies – an approach that I think is particularly useful for developing systematic reviews in healthcare policy making.[50,51] But these relatively small-print applications are all beyond the basics, and if you're reading this book to get you through an exam, you'll probably find they aren't on the syllabus.

If you found yourself sympathising with Professor Eysenck in the previous section, you might like to look at some other theoretical critiques of systematic review. Maggie MacLure has written an excellent philosophical article claiming that with its overemphasis on protocols and procedures, conventional systematic review degrades the status of interpretive scholarly activities such as reading, writing and talking, and replaces them with a series of auditable technical tasks.[52] This change, she claims, is partly driven by the new managerialism in research and results in 'the call-centre version of research synthesis'. Her views are echoed by Loke, who argues that the focus on technical precisions strips so much meaning out of the research being reported that systematic reviews are virtually unreadable.[53] My own view is that while MacLure and Loke have a point, we shouldn't throw the baby out with the bath water. Systematic review, in its place, saves lives.

References

1 Caveman A. The invited review? Or, my field, from my standpoint, written by me using only my data and my ideas, and citing only my publications. *J Cell Sci* 2000;**113**:3125–6.

2 Knipschild P. Some examples of systematic reviews. In: Chalmers I, Altman D, eds. *Systematic reviews*. London: BMJ Publications, 1995.

3 Pauling L. *How to live longer and feel better*. New York: Freeman, 1986.

4 Mulrow CD. The medical review article: state of the science. *Ann Intern Med* 1987;**106**:485–8.

5 McAlister FA, Clark HD, van Walraven C, Straus SE, Lawson FM, Moher D *et al.* The medical review article revisited: has the science improved? *Ann Intern Med* 1999;**131**:947–51.

6 Oxman AD, Guyatt GH. The science of reviewing research. *Ann N Y Acad Sci* 1993;**703**:125–33.

7 Antman EM, Lau J, Kupelnick B, Mosteller F, Chalmers TC. A comparison of results of meta-analyses of randomized control trials and recommendations of clinical experts. Treatments for myocardial infarction. *JAMA* 1992;**268**:240–8.

8 Moher D, Cook DJ, Eastwood S, Olkin I, Rennie D, Stroup DF. Improving the quality of reports of meta-analyses of randomised controlled trials: the QUOROM statement. Quality of Reporting of Meta-analyses. *Lancet* 1999;**354**:1896–900.

9 Saxena R, Koudstaal P. Anticoagulants versus antiplatelet therapy for preventing stroke in patients with nonrheumatic atrial fibrillation and a history of stroke or transient ischemic attack. *Cochrane Database Syst Rev* 2004;CD000187.

10 Greenhalgh T, Robert G, Macfarlane F, Bate P, Kyriakidou O. Diffusion of innovations in service organisations: systematic literature review and recommendations for future research. *Millbank Q* 2004;**82**:581–629.

11 Moher D, Pham B, Klassen TP, Schulz KF, Berlin JA, Jadad AR *et al.* What contributions do languages other than English make on the results of meta-analyses? *J Clin Epidemiol* 2000;**53**:964–72.

12 Greenhalgh T, Peacock R. What are the most efficient search methods in systematic reviews of complex evidence? An audit of 495 primary sources. *BMJ* 2006 (in press).

13 Knipschild P. Searching for alternatives: loser pays. *Lancet* 1993;**341**:1135–6.

14 *Cochrane reviewers' handbook 4.2.2.* Chichester: John Wiley & Sons Ltd, 2004.

15 Atkins D, Eccles M, Flottorp S, Guyatt GH, Henry D, Hill S *et al.* Systems for grading the quality of evidence and the strength of recommendations I: critical appraisal of existing approaches The GRADE Working Group. *BMC Health Serv Res* 2004;**4**(1):38.

16 Atkins D, Briss PA, Eccles M, Flottorp S, Guyatt GH, Harbour RT *et al.* Systems for grading the quality of evidence and the strength of recommendations II: pilot study of a new system. *BMC Health Serv Res* 2005;**5**(1):25.

17 Balk EM, Bonis PA, Moskowitz H, Schmid CH, Ioannidis JP, Wang C *et al.* Correlation of quality measures with estimates of treatment effect in meta-analyses of randomized controlled trials. *JAMA* 2002;**287**:2973–82.

18 Counsell CE, Clarke MJ, Slattery J, Sandercock PA. The miracle of DICE therapy for acute stroke: fact or fictional product of subgroup analysis? *BMJ* 1994;**309**:1677–81.

19 Grimley Evans J. Evidence-based and evidence-biased medicine. *Age Ageing* 1995;**24**:461–3.

20 Fergusson D, Glass K, Hutton B, Shapiro S. Randomised controlled trials of aprotinin in cardiac surgery: could clinical equipoise have stopped the bleeding? *Clin Trials* 2005;**2**:218–32.

21 Pocock SJ, Henderson RA, Rickards AF, Hampton JR, King SB, III, Hamm CW *et al.* Meta-analysis of randomised trials comparing coronary angioplasty with bypass surgery. *Lancet* 1995;**346**:1184–9.

22 Chalmers I, Altman D, Egger M, Davey Smith G. *Systematic reviews in health care: meta-analysis in context*. London: BMJ Publications, 2001.

23 Egger M, Smith GD, Phillips AN. Meta-analysis: principles and procedures. *BMJ* 1997;**315**:1533–7.

24 Stewart LA, Tierney JF. To IPD or not to IPD? Advantages and disadvantages of systematic reviews using individual patient data. *Eval Health Prof* 2002;**25**: 76–97.

25 Egger M, Smith GD. Meta-analysis. Potentials and promise. *BMJ* 1997;**315**: 1371–4.

26 Egger M, Schneider M, Davey SG. Meta-analysis. Spurious precision? Meta-analysis of observational studies. *BMJ* 1998;**316**:140–4.

27 Egger M, Smith GD. Meta-analysis. Bias in location and selection of studies. *BMJ* 1998;**316**:61–6.

28 Davey SG, Egger M, Phillips AN. Meta-analysis. Beyond the grand mean? *BMJ* 1997;**315**:1610–14.

29 Davey SG, Egger M. Meta-analysis. Unresolved issues and future developments. *BMJ* 1998;**316**:221–5.

30 Egger M, Smith GD, Sterne JA. Uses and abuses of meta-analysis. *Clin Med* 2001;**1**:478–84.

31 Egger M, Ebrahim S, Smith GD. Where now for meta-analysis? *Int J Epidemiol* 2002;**31**:1–5.

32 Thompson SG. Why and how sources of heterogeneity should be investigated. In: Egger M, Davey Smith G, Altman DG, eds. *Systematic reviews in health care: meta-analysis in context*. London: BMJ Publications, 2001.

33 Eysenck HJ. Problems with meta-analysis. In: Chalmers I, Altman DG, eds. *Systematic reviews*. London: BMJ Publications, 1995.

34 Higgins JP, Spiegelhalter DJ. Being sceptical about meta-analyses: a Bayesian perspective on magnesium trials in myocardial infarction. *Int J Epidemiol* 2002;**31**:96–104.

35 Egger M, Smith GD. Misleading meta-analysis: lessons from 'an effective, safe, simple' intervention that wasn't. *BMJ* 1995;**311**:753–4.

36 LeLorier J, Gregoire G, Benhaddad A, Lapierre J, Derderian F. Discrepancies between meta-analyses and subsequent large randomized, controlled trials. *N Engl J Med* 1997;**337**:536–42.

37 Griffin S. Diabetes care in general practice: meta-analysis of randomised control trials. *BMJ* 1998;**317**:390–6.

38 Greenhalgh T. Commentary: meta-analysis is a blunt and potentially misleading instrument for analysing models of service delivery. *BMJ* 1998;**317**:395–6.

39 Egger M, Davey Smith G. Systematic reviews of observational studies. In: Egger M, Davey Smith G, Altman DG, eds. *Systematic reviews in health care: meta-analysis in context*, London: BMJ Publications, 2001.

40 Norris SL, Atkins D. Challenges in using nonrandomized studies in systematic reviews of treatment interventions. *Ann Intern Med* 2005;**142**:1112–19.

41 Chou R, Helfand M. Challenges in systematic reviews that assess treatment harms. *Ann Intern Med* 2005;**142**:1090–9.

42 Deeks J. Systematic reviews of evaluations of diagnostic and screening tests. In: Egger M, Davey Smith G, Altman DG, eds. *Systematic reviews in health care: meta-analysis in context*. London: BMJ Publications, 2001.

43 Tatsioni A, Zarin DA, Aronson N, Samson DJ, Flamm CR, Schmid C *et al*. Challenges in systematic reviews of diagnostic technologies. *Ann Intern Med* 2005;**142**:1048–55.

44 Shekelle PG, Morton SC, Suttorp MJ, Buscemi N, Friesen C. Challenges in systematic reviews of complementary and alternative medicine topics. *Ann Intern Med* 2005;**142**:1042–7.

45 Reed D, Price EG, Windish DM, Wright SM, Gozu A, Hsu EB *et al*. Challenges in systematic reviews of educational intervention studies. *Ann Intern Med* 2005;**142**:1080–9.

46 Mugford M. Using systematic reviews for economic evaluation. In: Egger M, Davey Smith G, Altman DG, eds. *Systematic reviews in health care: meta-analysis in context*. London: BMJ Publications, 2001.

47 Pignone M, Saha S, Hoerger T, Lohr KN, Teutsch S, Mandelblatt J. Challenges in systematic reviews of economic analyses. *Ann Intern Med* 2005;**142**:1073–9.

48 Thomas J, Harden A, Oakley A, Oliver S, Sutcliffe K, Rees R *et al*. Integrating qualitative research with trials in systematic reviews. *BMJ* 2004;**328**:1010–12.

49 Dixon-Woods M, Agarwal S, Jones D, Young B, Sutton A. Synthesising qualitative and quantitative evidence: a review of possible methods. *J Health Serv Res Policy* 2005;**10**:45–53.

50 Pawson R, Greenhalgh T, Harvey G, Walshe K. Realist review – a new method of systematic review designed for complex policy interventions. *J Health Serv Res Policy* 2005;**10** (Suppl 1):21–34.

51 Greenhalgh T, Robert G, Macfarlane F, Bate P, Kyriakidou O, Peacock R. Storylines of research in diffusion of innovation: a meta-narrative approach to systematic review. *Soc Sci Med* 2005;**61**:417–30.

52 MacLure M. 'Clarity bordering on stupidity': where's the quality in systematic review? *J Educ Policy* 2005;**20**:393–416.

53 Loke YK, Derry S. Does anybody read 'evidence-based' articles? *BMC Med Res Methodol* 2003;**3**:14.

Chapter 9 **Papers that tell you what to do (guidelines)**

9.1 The great guidelines debate

Never was the chasm between front-line clinicians and back-room policy makers wider than in their respective attitudes to clinical guidelines. Policy makers (by which I include everyone who has a view on how medicine ought to be practised in an ideal world – including politicians, senior managers, clinical directors, academics and teachers) tend to love guidelines. Front-line clinicians (i.e. people who spend all their time seeing patients) very often have a strong aversion to guidelines.

Before we carry this political hot potato any further, we need a definition of guidelines, for which the following will suffice:

> Guidelines are systematically developed statements to assist
> practitioner decisions about appropriate health care for specific
> clinical circumstances

The best paper I've read recently on evidence-based guidelines (what they are, how they're developed, why we need them and what the controversies are) was published recently by one of my lecturers, Deborah Swinglehurst.[1] I have drawn extensively on her review when updating this chapter. One important distinction that Deborah makes in her paper is between guidelines (which are generally expressed in terms of general principles and leave room for judgement within broad parameters) and protocols, which she defines as follows:

> Protocols are instructions on what to do in particular circumstances.
> They are similar to guidelines but include less room for individual
> judgement, are often produced for less experienced staff, or for use in
> situations where eventualities are predictable.

> **Box 9.1** Purpose of guidelines
>
> 1 To make evidence-based standards explicit and accessible (but see below: few guidelines currently in circulation are truly evidence based).
> 2 To make decision making in the clinic and at the bedside easier and more objective.
> 3 To provide a yardstick for assessing professional performance.
> 4 To delineate the division of labour (e.g. between GPs and consultants).
> 5 To educate patients and professionals about 'current best practice'.
> 6 To improve the cost-effectiveness of health services.
> 7 To serve as a tool for external control.

The purposes that guidelines serve are given in Box 9.1. Clinician resistance to guidelines has a number of explanations.[2–8] These include

1 Clinical freedom ('I'm not having anyone telling me how to manage my patients').
2 Debates amongst experts about the quality of evidence ('Well, if they can't agree among themselves …').
3 Lack of appreciation of evidence by practitioners ('That's all very well, but when I trained we were always taught to hold back on steroids for asthma').
4 Defensive medicine ('I'll check all the tests anyway – belt and braces').
5 Strategic and cost constraints ('We can't afford to replace the equipment').
6 Specific practical constraints ('Where on earth did I put those guidelines'?).
7 Failure of patients to accept procedures ('Mrs Brown insists she only needs a smear every 5 years').
8 Competing influences of other non-medical factors ('When we get the new computer system up and running …').
9 Lack of appropriate, patient-specific feedback on performance ('I seem to be treating this condition OK').

The image of the medical buffoon blundering blithely through the outpatient clinic still diagnosing the same illnesses and prescribing the same drugs he (or she) learnt about at medical school 40 years previously, and never having read a paper since, knocks the 'clinical freedom' argument right out of the arena. Such hypothetical situations are grist to the mill of those who would impose 'expert guidelines' on most if not all medical practice and hold to account all those who fail to keep in step.

But the counter-argument to the excessive use, and particularly the compulsive imposition, of clinical guidelines is a powerful one, and it has been expressed very eloquently by Professor Sir John Grimley Evans:

> There is a fear that in the absence of evidence clearly applicable to the case in the hand a clinician might be forced by guidelines to make use of evidence which is only doubtfully relevant, generated perhaps in a different grouping of patients in another country at some other time and using a similar but not identical treatment. This is evidence-biased medicine; it is to use evidence in the manner of the fabled drunkard who searched under the street lamp for his door key because that is where the light was, even though he had dropped the key somewhere else.[9]

Grimley Evans's fear, which every practising clinician shares but few can articulate, is that politicians and health service managers who have jumped on the evidence-based medicine bandwagon will use guidelines to decree the treatment of diseases rather than of patients. They will, it is feared, make judgements about people and their illnesses subservient to published evidence that an intervention is effective 'on average'. This, and other real and perceived disadvantages of guidelines, are given in Box 9.2, which has been compiled from a number of sources.[1–8,10] But if you read the distinction between guidelines and protocols above, you will probably have realised that

---

Box 9.2 Drawbacks of guidelines (real and perceived)

1 Guidelines may be intellectually suspect and reflect 'expert opinion', which may formalise unsound practice.

2 By reducing medical practice variation they may standardise to 'average' rather than best practice.

3 They might inhibit innovation and prevent individual cases from being dealt with discretely and sensitively.

4 Guidelines developed at national or regional level may not reflect local needs or have the 'ownership' of local practitioners.

5 Guidelines developed in secondary care may not reflect demographic, clinical or practical differences between this setting and the primary care setting.

6 Guidelines may produce undesirable shifts in the balance of power between different professional groups (e.g. between clinicians and academics or purchasers and providers). Hence, guideline development may be perceived as a political act.

7 Out-of-date guidelines might hold back the implementation of new research evidence.

a good guideline wouldn't 'force' you to abandon common sense or judgement – it would simply flag up a recommended course of action for you to consider. Nevertheless, even a perfect guideline can make work for the busy clinician. My friend Neal Maskrey recently sent me this quote from an article in the *Lancet*:

'We surveyed one [24-h] acute medical take in our hospital. In a relatively quiet take, we saw 18 patients with a total of 44 diagnoses. The guidelines that the on call physician should have read remembered and applied correctly for those conditions came to 3679 pages. This number included only NICE [UK National Institute for Health and Clinical Excellence], the Royal Colleges and major societies from the last 3 years. If it takes 2 min to read each page, the physician on call will have to spend 122h reading to keep abreast of the guidelines.[11]

The mushrooming guidelines industry owes its success at least in part to a growing 'accountability culture' that is now (many argue) being set in statute in many countries. In the UK National Health Service, all doctors, nurses, pharmacists and other health professions now have a contractual duty to provide clinical care based on best available research evidence.[12] Officially produced or sanctioned guidelines – such as those produced by the UK National Institute of Clinical Excellence www.nice.org.uk or linked via the National Electronic Library for Health Guidelines Finder NELH Guidelines finder http://libraries.nelh.nhs.uk/guidelinesFinder/ – are a way of both supporting and policing that laudable goal. While the medicolegal implications of 'official' guidelines have rarely been tested in the United Kingdom,[13] courts in North America have ruled that guideline developers can be held liable for faulty guidelines.[14] More worryingly, a U.S. court recently refused to accept adherence to an evidence-based guideline (which advised doctors to share the inherent uncertainty associated with PSA testing in asymptomatic middle-aged men, and make a shared decision on whether the test was worth doing) as defence by a doctor being sued for missing an early prostate cancer in an unlucky 53 year old.[15]

9.2 How can we help ensure that evidence-based guidelines are followed?

Two of the leading international authorities on the thorny topic of implementation of clinical guidelines are Richard Grol and Jeremy Grimshaw. In one early study by Grol's team, the main factors associated with successfully

Table 9.1 Classification of clinical guidelines in terms of probability of being effective, reproduced from Grimshaw and Russell.[14]

Probability of being effective	Development strategy	Dissemination strategy	Implementation strategy
High	Internal	Specific educational intervention (e.g. problem-based learning package)	Patient-specific reminder at time of consultation
Above average	Intermediate	Continuing education (e.g. lecture)	Patient-specific feedback
Below average	External, local	Mailing targeted groups	General feedback
Low	External, national	Publication in journal	General reminder

following a guideline or protocol were the practitioners' perception that it was uncontroversial (68% compliance versus 35% if it was perceived to be controversial), evidence based (71% versus 57% if not), contained explicit recommendations (67% versus 36% if the recommendations were vague) and required no change to existing routines (67% versus 44% if a major change was recommended).[16]

An early paper by Grimshaw and Russell,[17] summarised in Table 9.1, showed that the probability of a guideline being effectively followed depended on three factors:

1 the development strategy (where and how the guideline was produced);
2 the dissemination strategy (how it was brought to the attention of clinicians); and
3 the implementation strategy (how the clinician was prompted and supported to follow the guideline, including organisational issues).

In terms of the development strategy, as Table 9.1 shows, the most effective guidelines are developed locally by the people who are going to use them, introduced as part of a specific educational intervention, and implemented via a patient-specific prompt that appears at the time of the consultation. The importance of ownership (i.e. the feeling by those being asked to play by new rules that they have been involved in drawing up those rules) is surely self-evident. There is also an extensive management theory literature to support the common sense notion that professionals will oppose changes that they perceive as threatening to their livelihood (i.e. income), self-esteem, sense of competence or autonomy. It stands to reason, therefore, that involving health professionals in setting the standards against which they are going to be judged generally produces greater changes in patient outcomes than occur if they are not involved.[18]

Grimshaw's conclusions from this early paper were initially misinterpreted by some people as implying that there was no place for nationally developed guidelines, since only locally developed ones had any impact. In fact, while local adoption and ownership is undoubtedly crucial to the success of a guideline programme, local teams produce more robust guidelines if they draw on the range of national and international resources of evidence-based recommendations and use this as their starting point.[19,20]

Input from local teams is not about reinventing the wheel in terms of summarising the evidence, but to take account of local practicalities when operationalising the guideline. For example, a nationally produced guideline about epilepsy care might recommend an epilepsy specialist nurse in every district. But in one district, the health care teams might have advertised for such a nurse but failed to recruit one. So the 'local input' might be about how best to provide what the epilepsy nurse would have provided, in the absence of a person in post.

In terms of dissemination and implementation of guidelines, Grimshaw's team published a comprehensive systematic review of strategies intended to improve doctors' implementation of guidelines in 2004,[21] and Grol and Grimshaw helpfully summarised this weighty tome in a joint review article for the *Lancet*.[22] The scope of the review and the primary studies are summarised in Box 9.3.

The findings confirmed the general principle that clinicians are not easily influenced, but that efforts to increase guideline use are often effective to some extent. Specifically:

1 Improvements were shown in the intended direction of the intervention in 86% of comparisons – but the effect was generally small in magnitude;
2 Simple reminders were the intervention most consistently observed to be effective;
3 Educational outreach programmes (e.g. visiting doctors in their clinics) only led to modest effects on implementation success – and were very expensive compared with less intensive approaches;
4 Dissemination of educational materials led to modest but potentially important effects (and of similar magnitude to more intensive interventions);
5 Multifaceted interventions were not necessarily more effective than single interventions;
6 Nothing could be concluded from most primary studies about the cost-effectiveness of the intervention.

Box 9.3 The Grimshaw *et al.* systematic review of guideline dissemination and implementation

What did the review cover?

1 Scope: primary studies testing guideline dissemination and implementation strategies.

2 Study designs: experimental or quasi-experimental study designs (randomised controlled trials, non-randomised controlled trials, controlled before and after studies and interrupted time series studies)*.

3 Participants: medically qualified health care professionals.

4 Interventions: guideline dissemination and implementation strategies.

5 Outcomes: objective measures of provider behaviour and/or patient outcome.

What were the primary studies?

Single interventions

    84 comparisons evaluated a single intervention against no intervention control including:

• 38 studies of reminders
• 18 studies of educational materials
• 12 studies of audit and feedback
• 3 studies of educational meetings
• 3 of 'other professional interventions'
• 2 studies of organisational interventions
• 8 studies of patient mediated interventions.

Multifaceted interventions

    138 comparisons against a 'no intervention' control group
• evaluated 68 different combinations of interventions
• maximum number of comparisons of same combination of interventions was 11.

    85 comparisons against an intervention control group
• evaluated 58 different combinations of interventions.

See text for a summary of the main findings.

* The authors have discussed choice of design from a theoretical perspective in separate commentary articles.[5,6]

The 2004 review reversed some previous 'received wisdom', which was probably the result of publication bias in trials of implementation strategies. Contrary to what I said in the first and second editions of this book, for example, expensive complex interventions aimed at improving the implementation of guidelines by doctors are generally no more effective than simple, cheaper, well-targeted ones.

Only 27% of the intervention studies reviewed by Grimshaw's team were considered to be based (either implicitly or explicitly) on a coherent theory of change – in other words, the researchers in such studies generally did not base the design of their intervention on a properly articulated mechanism of action ('A is intended to lead to B which is intended to lead to C'). In a separate paper, his team argues strongly that research into implementing guidelines should become more theory driven.[23]

One of Grimshaw's most important contributions to EBM was to set up a special subgroup of the Cochrane Collaboration (see Section 2.10) to review and summarise emerging research on the use of guidelines and other related issues in improving professional practice.[24] You can find details of the Effective Practice and Organisation of Care (EPOC) Group on the Cochrane website (www.epoc.uottawa.ca). The EPOC database now lists over 3000 primary studies on the general theme of getting research evidence into practice.

For an accessible if slightly out-of-date discussion on the barriers to implementing guidelines, see the *BMJ*'s 1999 series.[4,19,25] In a nutshell, the successful introduction of guidelines needs 'careful attention to the principles of change management: in particular, . . . leadership, energy, avoidance of unnecessary uncertainty, good communication, and, above all, time'.[26] See also my own summary of how to influence the practice of clinicians in Chapter 13.

It's also worth looking at the paper by Grol entitled 'Beliefs and evidence in changing clinical practice'.[27] In it, he depicts a typical scene of guideline implementation in which different stakeholders have different views and approaches. Researchers want to do randomised controlled trials of interventions; educationists want to develop a robust training programme for the clinicians; financiers want something that stays within budget; and organisational theorists generally want to develop a 'system-wide' strategy. Grol rightly concludes that there is no quick fix for the complex challenge of getting the patient to receive the right management from the right clinician at the right time.

If you're interested in reading more about the messy world of implementing guidelines at the level of health care policy, see Jonathan Lomas's superb monograph 'Beyond the sound of one hand clapping'.[28] Michie and Johnston recently published a review that demonstrated that a guideline recommending a specific course of action is more likely to be implemented than one suggesting a vague direction of action![2] Finally, for an overview of the challenges faced when guideline implementation requires major organisational-level innovation (e.g. when a hospital must invest in a major new piece of equipment or drastically revise the job descriptions of key staff), see the systematic review by my own team.[29]

9.3 Ten questions to ask about a clinical guideline

Deborah Swinglehurst rightly points out that all the song and dance about encouraging clinicians to follow guidelines is only justified if the guideline is worth following in the first place.[1] Sadly, not all of them are. She suggests two aspects of a good guideline – the content (e.g. whether it is based on a comprehensive and rigorous systematic review of the evidence) and the process (how the guideline was put together). I would add a third aspect – the presentation of the guideline (how appealing it is to the busy clinician and how easy it is to follow).

Like all published articles, guidelines would be easier to evaluate on all these counts if they were presented in a standardised format, and an international standard (the AGREE instrument) for developing, reporting and presenting guidelines was recently published.[30] Box 9.4 offers a pragmatic checklist, based partly on the work of the AGREE group, for structuring your assessment of a clinical guideline; and Box 9.5 reproduces the AGREE criteria in full. Since few published guidelines currently follow such a format, you will probably have to scan the full text for answers to the questions below. In preparing this list I have drawn on a number of previously published articles as well as the relatively new AGREE instrument.[2,20,30–34]

Question 1: did the preparation and publication of this guideline involve a significant conflict of interest?

I will resist labouring the point, but a drug company that makes hormone replacement therapy, or a research professor whose life's work has been spent perfecting this treatment, might be tempted to recommend it for wider indications than the average clinician. Much has been written about the 'medicalisation' of human experience (are energetic children with a short attention span 'hyperactive'?; should women with low sex drive be offered 'treatment' – and so on). A guideline may be evidence based, but the problem it addresses will have been constructed by a team that views the world in a particular way.

Question 2: is the guideline concerned with an appropriate topic, and does it state clearly the target group it applies to?

Key questions in relation to choice of topic, reproduced from an article published a few years ago in the *British Medical Journal*,[35] are given in Box 9.6.

Box 9.4 Checklist for assessing a clinical guideline

1 *Objective*: the primary objective of the guideline, including the health problem and the targeted patients, providers and settings.

2 *Options*: the clinical practice options considered in formulating the guideline.

3 *Outcomes*: significant health and economic outcomes considered in comparing alternative practices.

4 *Evidence*: how and when evidence was gathered, selected and synthesised.

5 *Values*: disclosure of how values were assigned to potential outcomes of practice options and who participated in the process.

6 *Benefits, harms and costs*: the type and magnitude of benefits, arms and costs expected for patients from guideline implementation.

7 *Recommendations*: summary of key recommendations.

8 *Validation*: report of any external review, comparison with other guidelines or clinical testing of guideline use.

9 *Sponsors and stakeholders*: disclosure of the persons who developed, funded or endorsed the guideline.

The Grimley Evans quote on p.136 begs the question 'To whom does this guideline apply'?. If the evidence related to people aged 18–65 with no comorbidity (i.e. with nothing else wrong with them except the disease being considered), it might not apply to your patient. Sometimes this means you will need to reject it outright, but more commonly, you will have to exercise your judgement in assessing its transferability.

Question 3: did the guideline development panel include *both* an expert in the topic area *and* a specialist in the methods of secondary research (e.g. meta-analyst, health economist)?
If a clinical guideline has been prepared entirely by a panel of internal 'experts', you should, paradoxically, look at it particularly critically since researchers have been shown to be less objective in appraising evidence in their own field of expertise than in someone else's.[36] The involvement of an outsider (an expert in guideline development rather than in the particular clinical topic) to act as arbiter and methodological adviser will, hopefully, make the process more objective. But as John Gabbay and his team recently showed in an elegant qualitative study, the hard-to-measure expertise (what might be called 'embodied knowledge') of front-line clinicians (in this case, general practitioners) contributed crucially to the development of workable local guidelines.[37]

Box 9.5 The six domains of the AGREE instrument (see reference 24)

Domain 1: Scope and purpose
1 The overall objective(s) of the guideline is (are) specifically described
2 The clinical question(s) covered by the guideline is (are) specifically described
3 The patients to whom the guideline is meant to apply are specifically described.

Domain 2: Stakeholder involvement
1 The guideline development group includes individuals from all the relevant professional groups
2 The patients' views and preferences have been sought
3 The target users of the guideline are clearly defined
4 The guideline has been piloted among end-users.

Domain 3: Rigour of development
1 Systematic methods were used to search for evidence
2 The criteria for selecting the evidence are clearly described
3 The methods used for formulating the recommendations are clearly described
4 The health benefits, side effects and risks have been considered in formulating the recommendations
5 There is an explicit link between the recommendations and the supporting evidence
6 The guideline has been externally reviewed by experts prior to its publication
7 A procedure for updating the guideline is provided.

Domain 4: Clarity and presentation
1 The recommendations are specific and unambiguous
2 The different options for management of the condition are clearly presented
3 Key recommendations are easily identifiable
4 The guideline is supported with tools for application.

Domain 5: Applicability
1 Potential organisational barriers in applying the recommendations have been discussed
2 Potential cost implications of applying the recommendations have been considered
3 The guideline presents key review criteria for monitoring and/or audit purposes.

Box 9.5 (Continued)

Domain 6: Editorial independence
1 The guideline is editorially independent from the funding body
2 Conflicts of interest of guideline development members have been
  recorded.

Box 9.6 Key questions on choice of topic for guideline development (see
reference 30)

- Is the topic high volume, high risk, high cost?
- Are there large or unexplained variations in practice?
- Is the topic important in terms of the process and outcome of patient care?
- Is there potential for improvement?
- Is the investment of time and money likely to be repaid?
- Is the topic likely to hold the interest of team members?
- Is consensus likely?
- Will change benefit patients?
- Can change be implemented?

Question 4: have the subjective judgements of the development panel been made explicit, and are they justified?

Guideline development is not just a technical process of finding evidence,
appraising it and turning it into recommendations. Recommendations also
require judgements (relating to personal or social values, ethical principles
and so on). As the UK National Institute for Health and Clinical Excellence
(NICE) has recently stated (see www.nice.org.uk), it is right and proper for
guideline developers to take account of the 'ethical principles, preferences,
culture and aspirations that should underpin the nature and extent of care
provided by the National Health Service'. Deborah Swinglehurst suggests four
sub-questions to ask about these subjective judgements:[1]

1 What *guiding principles* have been used to decide how effective an intervention must be (compared to its potential harms) before its recommendation
   is considered?
2 What *values* have underpinned the panel's decisions about which guideline
   developments to prioritise?
3 What is the *ethical framework* to which guideline developers are working –
   in particular relating to matters of distributive justice ('rationing')?
4 Where there was disagreement between guideline developers, what *explicit
   processes* have been used to resolve such disagreements?

Question 5: have all the relevant data been scrutinised and rigorously evaluated?

The academic validity of guidelines depends (among other things) on whether they are supported by high-quality primary research studies, and on how strong the evidence from these studies is. At the most basic level, was the literature analysed at all, or are these guidelines simply a statement of the preferred practice of a selected panel of experts (i.e. consensus guidelines)? If the literature was looked at, was a systematic search done, and if so, did it broadly follow the method described in Section 8.2? Were all papers unearthed by the search included, or was an explicit scoring system (such as GRADE[34]) used to reject those of poor methodological quality and give those of high quality the extra weight they deserved?

Of course, up-to-date systematic reviews should ideally be the raw material for guideline development. But in many cases, a search for rigorous and relevant research on which to base guidelines proves fruitless, and the authors, unavoidably, resort to 'best available' evidence or expert opinion.

Question 6: has the evidence been properly synthesised, and are the guideline's conclusions in keeping with the data on which they are based?

Another key determinant of the validity of a guideline is how the different studies contributing to it have been pulled together (i.e. synthesised) in the context of the clinical and policy needs being addressed. For one thing, a systematic review and meta-analysis might have been appropriate, and if the latter, issues of probability and confidence should have been dealt with acceptably (see Section 4.7).

But systematic reviews don't exist (and never will exist) to cover every eventuality in clinical decision making and policy making. In many areas, especially complex ones, the opinion of experts is still the best 'evidence' around, and in such cases guideline developers should adopt rigorous methods to ensure that it isn't just the voice of the expert who talks for longest in the meetings that drives the recommendations. Paul Shekelle from the RAND Corporation in the United States has undertaken some exciting research into methods for improving the rigour of consensus recommendations so as to ensure, for example, that an appropriate mix of experts is chosen, everyone reads the available research evidence, everyone gets an equal vote, all points of contention (raised anonymously) are fully discussed, and the resulting recommendations indicate the extent of agreement and dissent between the panel.[19,38] The UK Health Technology Assessment Programme has produced a valuable overview of the strengths and limitations of consensus methods which is available in full text on the Internet.[39]

Question 7: does the guideline address variations in medical practice and other controversial areas (e.g. optimum care in response to genuine or perceived underfunding)?

It would be foolish to make dogmatic statements about ideal practice without reference to what actually goes on in the real world. There are many instances where some practitioners are marching to an altogether different tune from the rest of us (see Section 1.2), and a good guideline should face such realities head on rather than hoping that the misguided minority will fall into step by default.

Another thorny issue which guidelines should tackle head-on is where essential compromises should be made if financial constraints preclude 'ideal' practice. If the ideal, for example, is to offer all patients with significant coronary artery disease a bypass operation (at the time of writing it isn't, but never mind), and the health service can only afford to fund 20% of such procedures, who should be pushed to the front of the queue?

Question 8: is the guideline clinically relevant, comprehensive and flexible?

In other words, is it written from the perspective of the practising doctor, nurse, midwife, physiotherapist and so on, and does it take into account the type of patients he or she is likely to see, and in what circumstances? Perhaps the most frequent source of trouble here is when guidelines developed in secondary care and intended for use in hospital outpatients (who tend to be at the sicker end of the clinical spectrum) are passed on to the primary health care team with the intention of their being used in the primary care setting, where, in general, patients are less ill and may well need fewer investigations and less aggressive management. This issue is discussed in Section 7.2 in relation to the different utility of diagnostic and screening tests in different populations.

Guidelines should cover all, or most, clinical eventualities. What if the patient is intolerant of the recommended medication? What if you can't send off all the recommended blood tests? What if the patient is very young, very old or suffers from a coexisting illness? These, after all, are the patients who prompt most of us to reach for our guidelines, while the more 'typical' patient tends to be managed without recourse to written instructions.

Flexibility is a particularly important consideration for national and regional bodies who set themselves up to develop guidelines. It has been repeatedly demonstrated that the ownership of guidelines by the people who are intended to use them locally is crucial to whether or not the guidelines are actually used.[17,21,40] If there is no free rein for practitioners to adapt them to meet local needs and priorities, a set of guidelines will probably never get taken out of the drawer.

Question 9: does the guideline take into account what is acceptable to, affordable by and practically possible for patients?

There is an apocryphal story of a physician in the 1940s (a time when no effective medicines for high blood pressure were available), who discovered that restricting the diet of hypertensive patients to plain, boiled, unsalted rice dramatically reduced their blood pressure and also reduced the risk of stroke. The story goes, however, that the diet made the patients so miserable that a lot of them committed suicide.

This is an extreme example, but within the past few years I have seen guidelines for treating constipation in the elderly that offered no alternative to the combined insults of large amounts of bran and twice daily suppositories. Small wonder that the district nurses who were issued with them (for whom I have a good deal of respect) have gone back to giving castor oil.

For a further discussion on how to incorporate the needs and priorities of patients in guideline development, see some recent reviews on consumer involvement in research.[41–43]

Question 10: does the guideline include recommendations for its own dissemination, implementation and regular review?

Given the well-documented gap between what is known to be good practice and what actually happens,[3,40,44,45] and the barriers to the successful implementation of guidelines discussed in Section 9.2, it would be in the interests of those who develop guidelines to suggest methods of maximising their use. If this objective were included as standard in the 'Guidelines for good guidelines', the guideline-writers' output would probably include fewer ivory tower recommendations and more that are plausible, possible and capable of being explained to patients. Having said that, one very positive development in evidence-based medicine since I wrote the first edition of this book is the change in guideline developers' attitudes: they now often take responsibility for linking their outputs to clinicians (and patients) in the real world and for reviewing and updating their recommendations periodically.

References

1 Swinglehurst D. Evidence-based guidelines: the theory and the practice. *Evid Based Med Public Health* 2005;**9**:308–14.

2 Michie S, Johnston M. Changing clinical behaviour by making guidelines specific. *BMJ* 2004;**328**:343–5.

3 Garfield FB, Garfield JM. Clinical judgment and clinical practice guidelines. *Int J Technol Assess Health Care* 2000;**16**:1050–60.

4 Feder G, Eccles M, Grol R, Griffiths C, Grimshaw J. Clinical guidelines: using clinical guidelines. *BMJ* 1999;**318**:728–30.

5 Grilli R, Trisolini R, Labianca R, Zola P. Evolution of physicians' attitudes towards practice guidelines. *J Health Serv Res Policy* 1999;**4**:215–19.

6 Lenfant C. Shattuck lecture – clinical research to clinical practice – lost in translation? *N Engl J Med* 2003;**349**:868–74.

7 Bassand JP, Priori S, Tendera M. Evidence-based vs. 'impressionist' medicine: how best to implement guidelines. *Eur Heart J* 2005;**26**:1155–8.

8 Hofer TP, Zemencuk JK, Hayward RA. When there is too much to do: how practicing physicians prioritize among recommended interventions. *J Gen Intern Med* 2004;**19**:646–53.

9 Grimley Evans J. Evidence-based and evidence-biased medicine. *Age Ageing* 1995;**24**:461–3.

10 Delamothe T. Wanted: guidelines that doctors will follow. *BMJ* 1993;**307**:218.

11 Allen D, Harkins KJ. Too much guidance? *Lancet* 2005;**365**:1768.

12 Secretary of State for Health. *A first class service: quality in the new NHS*. London: The Stationery Office, 1998.

13 Hurwitz B. How does evidence based guidance influence determinations of medical negligence? *BMJ* 2004;**329**:1024–8.

14 McDonagh RJ, Hurwitz B. Lying in the bed we've made: reflection on some unintended consequences of clinical practice guidelines in the courts. *J Obstet Gynaecol Can* 2003;**25**:139–43.

15 Merenstein D. A piece of my mind. Winners and losers. *JAMA* 2004;**291**:15–16.

16 Grol R, Dalhuijsen J, Thomas S, Veld C, Rutten G, Mokkink H. Attributes of clinical guidelines that influence use of guidelines in general practice: observational study. *BMJ* 1998;**317**:858–61.

17 Grimshaw J, Russell IT. Effect of clinical guidelines on medical practice. A systematic review of rigorous evaluations. *Lancet* 1993;**342**:1317–22.

18 Report from General Practice 26. *The development and implementation of clinical guidelines*. London: Royal College of General Practitioners, 1995.

19 Shekelle P, Woolf SH, Eccles MP, Grimshaw JM. Clinical guidelines: developing guidelines. *BMJ* 1999;**318**:593–6.

20 Burgers JS, Cluzeau FA, Hanna SE, Hunt C, Grol R. Characteristics of high-quality guidelines: evaluation of 86 clinical guidelines developed in ten European countries and Canada. *Int J Technol Assess Health Care* 2003;**19**:148–57.

21 Grimshaw JM, Thomas RE, MacLennan G, Fraser C, Ramsay CR, Vale L, Whitty P, Eccles MP, Matowe L, Shirran L, Wensing M, Dikstra R, Donaldson C and Hutchinson A. Effectiveness and efficiency of guideline dissemination and implementation strategies. *Health Technol Assess Rep* 2004;**8**:1–72.

22 Grol R, Grimshaw J. From best evidence to best practice: effective implementation of change in patients' care. *Lancet* 2003;**362**:1225–30.

23 Eccles M, Grimshaw J, Walker A, Johnston M, Pitts N. Changing the behavior of healthcare professionals: the use of theory in promoting the uptake of research findings. *J Clin Epidemiol* 2005;**58**:107–12.

24 Mowatt G, Grimshaw JM, Davis DA, Mazmanian PE. Getting evidence into practice: the work of the Cochrane Effective Practice and Organization of care Group (EPOC). *J Contin Educ Health Prof* 2001;**21**:55–60.

25 Woolf SH, Grol R, Hutchinson A, Eccles M, Grimshaw J. Clinical guidelines: potential benefits, limitations, and harms of clinical guidelines. *BMJ* 1999;**318**: 527–30.

26 Ayers P, Renvoize T, Robinson M. Clinical guidelines: key decisions for acute service providers. *Br J Health Care Manage* 1995;**1**:547–51.

27 Grol R. Personal paper. Beliefs and evidence in changing clinical practice. *BMJ* 1997;**315**:418–21.

28 Lomas J. Improving research dissemination and uptake in the health sector: beyond the sound of one hand clapping, Policy Commentary C97-1. McMaster University, Hamilton, Ontario: Centre for Health Economics and Policy Analysis, 1997.

29 Greenhalgh T, Robert G, Macfarlane F, Bate P, Kyriakidou O. Diffusion of innovations in service organisations: systematic literature review and recommendations for future research. *Millbank Q* 2004;**82**:581–629.

30 Development and validation of an international appraisal instrument for assessing the quality of clinical practice guidelines: the AGREE project. *Qual Saf Health Care* 2003;**12**:18–23.

31 Hayward RS, Wilson MC, Tunis SR, Bass EB, Guyatt G. Users' guides to the medical literature. VIII. How to use clinical practice guidelines. A. Are the recommendations valid? Evidence-Based Medicine Working Group. *JAMA* 1995;**274**:570–4.

32 Wilson MC, Hayward RS, Tunis SR, Bass EB, Guyatt G. Users' guides to the medical literature. VIII. How to use clinical practice guidelines. B. what are the recommendations and will they help you in caring for your patients? Evidence-Based Medicine Working Group. *JAMA* 1995;**274**:1630–2.

33 Schunemann HJ, Best D, Vist G, Oxman AD. Letters, numbers, symbols and words: how to communicate grades of evidence and recommendations. *CMAJ* 2003;**169**:677–80.

34 Atkins D, Eccles M, Flottorp S, Guyatt GH, Henry D, Hill S *et al.* Systems for grading the quality of evidence and the strength of recommendations I: critical appraisal of existing approaches. The GRADE Working Group. *BMC Health Serv Res* 2004;**4**(1):38.

35 Thomson R, Lavender M, Madhok R. How to ensure that guidelines are effective. *BMJ* 1995;**311**:237–42.

36 Cook DJ, Greengold NL, Ellrodt AG, Weingarten SR. The relation between systematic reviews and practice guidelines. *Ann Intern Med* 1997;**127**:210–16.

37 Gabbay J, le May A. Evidence based guidelines or collectively constructed 'mindlines?' Ethnographic study of knowledge management in primary care. *BMJ* 2004;**329**:1013–16.

38 Campbell SM, Hann M, Roland MO, Quayle JA, Shekelle PG. The effect of panel membership and feedback on ratings in a two-round Delphi survey: results of a randomized controlled trial. *Med Care* 1999;**37**:964–8.

39 Murphy MK, Black NA, Lamping DL, McKee CM, Sanderson CF, Askham J *et al*. Consensus development methods, and their use in clinical guideline development. *Health Technol Assess* 1998;**2**:i-88.

40 Granados A, Jonsson E, Banta HD, Bero L, Bonair A, Cochet C *et al*. EUR-ASSESS project subgroup report on dissemination and Impact. *Int J Technol Assess Health Care* 1997;**13**:220–86.

41 Boote J, Telford R, Cooper C. Consumer involvement in health research: a review and research agenda. *Health Policy* 2002;**61**:213–36.

42 Oliver S, Clarke-Jones L, Rees R, Milne R, Buchanan P, Gabbay G, Gyte G, Oakley A, Stein K. Involving consumers in research and development agenda setting for the NHS: developing and evidence-based approach. *Health Technol Assess* 2004;**8**(15):1–148.

43 van Wersch A, Eccles M. Involvement of consumers in the development of evidence based clinical guidelines: practical experiences from the North of England evidence based guideline development programme. *Qual Health Care* 2001;**10**:10–16.

44 Buchan H. Gaps between best evidence and practice: causes for concern. *Med J Aust* 2004;**180**:S48–S49.

45 van Weel C. Translating research into practice – a three-paper series. *Lancet* 2003;**362**:1170.

Chapter 10 **Papers that tell you what things cost (economic analyses)**

10.1 What is economic analysis?

An economic analysis can be defined as *one that involves the use of analytical techniques to define choices in resource allocation*. Most of what I have to say on this subject comes from advice prepared by Professor Michael Drummond's team for authors and reviewers of economic analyses[1] and three of the Users' Guides to the Medical Literature series,[2–4] as well as the excellent pocket-sized summary by Jefferson *et al.*,[5] all of which emphasise the importance of setting the economic questions about a paper in the context of the overall quality and relevance of the study (see Section 10.3).

The first economic evaluation I ever remember was a TV advertisement in which the pop singer Cliff Richard tried to persuade a housewife that the most expensive brand of washing-up liquid on the market 'actually works out cheaper'. It was, apparently, stronger on stains, softer on the hands and produced more bubbles per penny than 'a typical cheap liquid'. Although I was only 9 at the time, I was unconvinced. Which 'typical cheap liquid' was the product being compared with? How much stronger on stains was it? Why should the effectiveness of a washing-up liquid be measured in terms of bubbles produced rather than plates cleaned?

Forgive me for sticking with this trivial example, but I'd like to use it to illustrate the four main types of economic evaluation which you will find in the literature (see Table 10.1 for the conventional definitions):

1 *cost-minimisation analysis:* '"Sudso" costs 47p per bottle whereas "Jiffo" costs 63p per bottle'.
2 *cost-effectiveness analysis:* '"Sudso" gives you 15 extra clean plates per wash than "Jiffo"'.
3 *cost–utility analysis:* 'In terms of quality-adjusted housewife hours (a composite score reflecting time and effort needed to scrub plates clean, and hand roughness caused by the liquid), "Sudso" provides 29 units per pound spent whereas "Jiffo" provides 23 units'.

Table 10.1 Types of economic analysis

Type of analysis	Outcome measure	Conditions of use	Example
Cost-minimisation analysis	No outcome measure	Used when the effect of both interventions is known (or may be assumed) to be identical	Comparing the price of a brand name drug with that of its generic equivalent if bioequivalence has been demonstrated
Cost-effectiveness analysis	Natural units (e.g. life-years gained)	Used when the effect of the interventions can be expressed in terms of one main variable	Comparing two preventive treatments for an otherwise fatal condition
Cost–utility analysis	Utility units (e.g. quality-adjusted life years)	Used when the effect of the interventions on health status has two or more important dimensions (e.g. benefits and side effects of drugs)	Comparing the benefits of two treatments for varicose veins in terms of surgical result, cosmetic appearance and risk of serious adverse event (e.g. pulmonary embolus)
Cost–benefit analysis	Monetary units (e.g. estimated cost of loss in productivity)	Used when it is desirable to compare an intervention for this condition with an intervention for a different condition	For a purchasing authority, to decide whether to fund a heart transplantation programme or a stroke rehabilitation ward

4 *cost–benefit analysis:* 'The net overall cost (reflecting direct cost of the product, indirect cost of time spent washing up, and estimated financial value of a clean plate relative to a slightly grubby one) of "Sudso" per day is 7.17p, while that of "Jiffo" is 9.32p'.

You should be able to see immediately that the most sensible analysis to use in this example is cost-effectiveness analysis. Cost-minimisation analysis (see Table 10.1) is inappropriate since 'Sudso' and 'Jiffo' do not have identical effectiveness. Cost–utility analysis is unnecessary since, in this example, we are interested in very little else apart from the number of plates cleaned per unit of washing-up liquid – in other words, our outcome has only one important dimension. Cost–benefit analysis is, in this example, an absurdly complicated way of telling you that 'Sudso' cleans more plates per penny.

There are, however, many situations where health professionals, particularly those who purchase health care from real cash-limited budgets, must choose between interventions for a host of different conditions whose outcomes (such as cases of measles prevented, increased mobility after a hip replacement, reduced risk of death from heart attack or likelihood of giving birth to a live baby) cannot be directly compared with one another. Controversy surrounds not just how these comparisons should be made (see Section 10.2), but also who should make them, and to whom the decision makers for the 'rationing' of health care should be accountable. These essential, fascinating and frustrating questions are beyond the scope of this book, but if you are interested I would recommend you look up the references listed at the end of this chapter.[5–14]

10.2 Measuring costs and benefits of health interventions

Not long ago, I was taken to hospital to have my appendix removed. From the hospital's point of view, the cost of my care included my board and lodging for 5 days, a proportion of doctors' and nurses' time, drugs and dressings, and investigations (blood tests and a scan). Other *direct costs* (see Box 10.1) included my general practitioner's time for attending me in the middle of the night, and the cost of the petrol my husband used when visiting me (not to mention the grapes and flowers).

In addition to this, there were the *indirect* costs of my loss in productivity. I was off work for 3 weeks, and my domestic duties were temporarily divided between various friends, neighbours and a nice young girl from a nanny agency. And, from my point of view, there were several *intangible* costs, such as discomfort, loss of independence, the allergic rash I developed on the medication and the cosmetically unsightly scar which I now carry on my abdomen.

As Box 10.1 shows, these direct, indirect and intangible costs constitute one side of the cost–benefit equation. On the benefit side, the operation greatly increased my chances of staying alive. In addition, I had a nice rest from work, and, to be honest, I rather enjoyed all the attention and sympathy. (Note that the 'social stigma' of appendicitis can be a positive one. I would be less likely to brag about my experience if my hospital admission had been precipitated by, say, an epileptic fit or a nervous breakdown, which have negative social stigmata.)

Box 10.1 Examples of costs and benefits of health interventions

Costs	Benefits
Direct	*Economic*
'Board and lodging'	Prevention of expensive-to-treat illness
Drugs, dressings, etc.	Avoidance of hospital admission
Investigations	Return to paid work
Staff salaries	
	Clinical
Indirect	Postponement of death or disability
Work days lost	Relief of pain, nausea, breathlessness, etc.
Value of 'unpaid' work	Improved vision, hearing, muscular strength, etc.
Intangible	*Quality of life*
Pain and suffering	Increased mobility and independence
Social stigma	Improved well-being
	Release from sick role

In the appendicitis example, few patients would perceive much freedom of choice in deciding to opt for the operation. But most health interventions do not concern definitive procedures for acutely life-threatening diseases. Most of us can count on developing at least one chronic, disabling and progressive condition such as ischaemic heart disease, high blood pressure, arthritis, chronic bronchitis, cancer, rheumatism, prostatic hypertrophy or diabetes. At some stage, almost all of us will be forced to decide whether having a routine operation, taking a particular drug or making a compromise in our lifestyle (reducing our alcohol intake or sticking to a cholesterol-lowering diet) is 'worth it'.

It is fine for informed individuals to make choices about their own care by gut reaction ('I'd rather live with my hernia than be cut open', or 'I know about the risk of thrombosis but I want to continue to smoke and stay on the Pill'). But when the choices are about other people's care, personal values and prejudices are the last thing that should enter the equation. Most of us would want the planners and policy makers to use objective, explicit and defensible criteria when making decisions such as, 'No, Mrs Brown may not have a kidney transplant'.

One important way of addressing the 'what's it worth?' question for a given health state (such as having poorly controlled diabetes or asthma) is to ask someone in that state how they feel. A number of questionnaires have been developed which attempt to measure overall health status, such as the Nottingham Health Profile, the SF-36 general health questionnaire (widely used in the United Kingdom) and the McMaster Health Utilities Index Questionnaire (popular in north America). For an overview of all these, see Ann Bowling's excellent book *Measuring Health*.[15]

In some circumstances, disease-specific measures of well-being are more valid than general measures. For example, answering 'yes' to the question, 'do you get very concerned about the food you are eating'? might indicate anxiety in someone without diabetes but normal self-care attitudes in someone with diabetes.[16] There has also been an upsurge of interest in *patient-specific* measures of quality of life, to allow different patients to place different values on particular aspects of their health and well-being. Of course, when quality of life is being analysed from the point of view of the patient, this is a sensible and humane approach. However, the health economist tends to make decisions about groups of patients or populations, in which case patient-specific, and even disease-specific, measures of quality of life have limited relevance. If you would like to get up to speed in the ongoing debate on how to measure health-related quality of life, take time to look up some of the references listed at the end of this chapter.[16–28]

The authors of standard instruments (such as the SF-36) for measuring quality of life have often spent years ensuring they are valid (i.e. they measure what we think they are measuring), reliable (they do so every time) and responsive to change (i.e. if an intervention improves or worsens the patient's health, the scale will reflect that). For this reason, you should be highly suspicious of a paper which eschews these standard instruments in favour of the authors' own rough-and-ready scale ('functional ability was classified as good, moderate or poor according to the clinician's overall impression', or, 'we asked patients to score both their pain and their overall energy level from one to ten, and added the results together'). Note also that even instruments which have apparently been well validated often do not stand up to rigorous evaluation of their psychometric validity.[17]

Another way of addressing the 'what's it worth'? of particular health states is through *health state preference values* – that is, the value which, in a hypothetical situation, a healthy person would place on a particular deterioration in their health, or which a sick person would place on a return to health. There are three main methods of assigning such values:[5,15,29]

1 *Rating scale measurements.* The respondent is asked to make a mark on a fixed line, labelled, for example, 'perfect health' at one end and 'death' at the other, to indicate where he or she would place the state in question (e.g. being wheelchair-bound from arthritis of the hip).

Box 10.2 Cost per QALY (see reference 30)

Cervical cancer screening	£200
Thrombolytic therapy following heart attack for men aged 35–39, compared with no therapy	£1,300
Thrombolytic therapy following heart attack for women aged 45–49, compared with no therapy	£2,000
Breast cancer screening (as per current U.K. protocol)	£6,800
Decreasing cervical cancer screening interval for women aged 20–59 from 5 to 3 years	£7,600
Coronary artery bypass graft for patients with mild angina and double vessel disease, compared with drug therapy	£26,000
Hospital dialysis for end-stage renal disease in people aged 55–64, compared with no treatment	£45,000

---

2 *Time trade-off measurements.* The respondent is asked to consider a particular health state (e.g. infertility) and estimate how many of their remaining years in full health they would sacrifice to be 'cured' of the condition.

3 *Standard gamble measurements.* The respondent is asked to consider the choice between living for the rest of their life in a particular health state and taking a 'gamble' (e.g. an operation) with a given odds of success which would return them to full health if it succeeded but kill them if it failed. The odds are then varied to see at what point the respondent decides the gamble is not worth taking.

The quality-adjusted life year (QALY) can be calculated by multiplying the preference value for that state with the time the patient is likely to spend in that state. The results of cost–benefit analyses are usually expressed in terms of 'cost per QALY', some examples of which are shown in Box 10.2.[30]

One of my many 'committee jobs' is sitting on the Appraisals Committee of NICE – the UK National Institute for Health and Clinical Excellence, which advises the Department of Health on the cost-effectiveness of medicines. It is very rare for the members of this multidisciplinary committee to get through a discussion on whether to recommend funding a controversial drug without major differences of opinion surfacing and emotions rising – and, in general, high-quality QALY data tend to generate light rather than heat in such discussions. Any measure of health state preference values is a reflection of the preferences and prejudices of the individuals who contributed to its development. Indeed, it is possible to come up with different values for QALYs depending on how the questions from which health state preference values are derived were posed.[31]

As medical ethicist John Harris has pointed out, QALYs are, like the society which produces them, inherently ageist, sexist, racist and loaded against those with permanent disabilities (since even a complete cure of an unrelated condition would not restore the individual to 'perfect health'). Furthermore, QALYs distort our ethical instincts by focusing our minds on life-years rather than people's lives. A disabled premature infant in need of an intensive care cot will, argues Harris, be allocated more resources than it deserves in comparison with a 50-year-old woman with cancer, since the infant, were it to survive, would have so many more life years to quality-adjust.[32]

There is an increasingly confusing array of alternatives to the QALY. Some of the ones that were in vogue when this book went to press include

1　Healthy Years Equivalent or HYE, a QALY-type measure that incorporates the individual's likely improvement or deterioration in health status in the future[33];

2　Willingness to Pay (WTP) or Willingness to Accept (WTA), measures of how much people would be prepared to pay to gain certain benefits or avoid certain problems[17,34,35];

3　Disability Adjusted Life Year or DALY, used mainly in the developing world to assess the overall burden of chronic disease and deprivation[36,37] – an increasingly used measure that is not without its critics[38]; and, perhaps most bizarrely

4　TWiST (time spent without symptoms of disease and toxicity of treatment) and Q-TWiST (quality-adjusted TWiST)![18]

My personal advice on all these measures is to look carefully at what goes into the number that is supposed to be an 'objective' indicator of a person's (or population's) health status, and at how the different measures might differ according to different disease states. In my view, they all have potential uses but none of them is an absolute or incontrovertible measure of health or illness! (Note, also, that I do not claim to be an expert on any of these measures or on how to calculate them – which is why I have offered a generous list of additional references at the end of this chapter.)

There is, however, another form of analysis which, although it does not abolish the need to place arbitrary numerical values on life and limb, avoids the buck stopping with the unfortunate health economist. This approach, known as *cost–consequences analysis*, presents the results of the economic analysis in a disaggregated form. In other words, it expresses different outcomes in terms of their different natural units (i.e. something real such as months of survival, legs amputated or take-home babies), so that individuals can assign their own values to particular health states before comparing two quite different interventions (e.g. infertility treatment versus cholesterol lowering, as in the example I mentioned in Chapter 1). Cost–consequences analysis allows for the health state preference values of both individuals and society to change with time, and is particularly useful when these are disputed or likely to change. This approach may also allow the analysis to be used by different groups or societies from the ones on which the original trial was performed.

10.3 Ten questions to ask about an economic analysis

The elementary checklist that follows is based largely on the sources mentioned in the first paragraph of this chapter. I strongly recommend that for a more definitive list, you check out these sources – especially the official recommendations by the BMJ working group.[1]

Question 1: is the analysis based on a study that answers a clearly defined clinical question about an economically important issue?

Before you attempt to digest what a paper says about costs, quality of life scales or utilities, make sure that the trial being analysed is scientifically relevant and capable of giving unbiased and unambiguous answers to the clinical question posed in its introduction (see Chapter 4). Furthermore, if there is clearly little to choose between the interventions in terms of either costs or benefits, a detailed economic analysis is probably pointless.

Question 2: from whose viewpoint are costs and benefits being considered?

From the patient's point of view, he or she generally wants to get better as quickly as possible. From the Treasury's point of view, the most cost-effective health intervention is one that returns all citizens promptly to taxpayer status and, when this status is no longer tenable, causes immediate sudden death. From the drug company's point of view, it would be difficult to imagine a cost–benefit equation that did not contain one of the company's products, and from a physiotherapist's point of view, the removal of a physiotherapy service would never be cost-effective. There is no such thing as an economic analysis which is devoid of perspective. Most assume the perspective of the health care system itself, although some take into account the hidden costs to the patient and society (e.g. due to work days lost). There is no 'right' perspective for an economic evaluation – but the paper should say clearly whose costs and whose benefits have been counted 'in' and 'out'.

Question 3: have the interventions being compared been shown to be clinically effective?

Nobody wants cheap treatment if it doesn't work. The paper you are reading may simply be an economic analysis, in which case it will based on a previously published clinical trial, or it will be an economic evaluation of a new trial whose clinical results are presented in the same paper. Either way, you must make sure that the intervention that 'works out cheaper' is not substantially less effective in clinical terms than the one that stands to be rejected on the grounds of cost. (Note, however, that in a resource-limited health care system, it is often very sensible to use treatments that are a little less effective when they are a lot less expensive than the best on offer!)

Question 4: are the interventions sensible and workable in the settings where they are likely to be applied?

A research trial that compares one obscure and unaffordable intervention with another will have little impact on medical practice. Remember that standard current practice (which may be 'doing nothing') should almost certainly be one of the alternatives compared. Too many research trials look at intervention packages that would be impossible to implement in the non-research setting (they assume, e.g. that general practitioners will own a state-of-the-art computer and agree to follow a protocol, that infinite nurse time is available for the taking of blood tests or that patients will make their personal treatment choices solely on the basis of the trial's primary outcome measure).

Question 5: which method of analysis was used, and was this appropriate?

This decision can be summarised as follows (see Section 10.2):

1 If the interventions produced identical outcomes $\Rightarrow$ cost-minimisation analysis.
2 If the important outcome is unidimensional $\Rightarrow$ cost-effectiveness analysis.
3 If the important outcome is multidimensional $\Rightarrow$ cost–utility analysis.
4 If the outcomes can be expressed meaningfully in monetary terms (i.e. if it is possible to weigh the cost–benefit equation for this condition against the cost–benefit equation for another condition) $\Rightarrow$ cost–benefit analysis.
5 If a cost–benefit analysis would otherwise be appropriate but the preference values given to different health states are disputed or likely to change $\Rightarrow$ cost–consequences analysis.

Question 6: how were costs and benefits measured?

Look back at Section 10.2, where I outlined some of the costs associated with my appendix operation. Now imagine a more complicated example – the rehabilitation of stroke patients into their own homes with attendance at a day centre compared with a standard alternative intervention (rehabilitation in a long-stay hospital). The economic analysis must take into account not just the time of the various professionals involved, the time of the secretaries and administrators who help run the service and the cost of the food and drugs consumed by the stroke patients, but also a fraction of the capital cost of building the day centre and maintaining a transport service to and from it.

There are no hard and fast rules for deciding which costs to include. If calculating 'cost per case' from first principles, remember that someone has to pay for heating, lighting, personnel support and even the accountants' bills of the institution. In general terms, these 'hidden costs' are known as overheads, and generally add an additional 30–60% onto the cost of a project. The task of costing things like operations and outpatient visits in the United Kingdom is easier than it used to be because these experiences are now bought and sold at a price that reflects (or should reflect) all overheads involved. Be warned, however, that unit costs of health interventions calculated in one country often bear no relation to those of the same intervention elsewhere, even when these costs are expressed as a proportion of GNP.

Benefits such as earlier return to work for a particular individual can, on the face of it, be measured in terms of the cost of employing that person at his or her usual daily rate. This approach has the unfortunate and politically unacceptable consequence of valuing the health of professional people higher than that of manual workers, homemakers or the unemployed, and that of the white majority higher than that of (generally) lower-paid minority ethnic groups. It might therefore be preferable to derive the cost of sick days from the average national wage.

In a cost-effectiveness analysis, changes in health status will be expressed in natural units (see Section 10.2). But just because the units are natural does not automatically make them appropriate. For example, the economic analysis of the treatment of peptic ulcer by two different drugs might measure outcome as 'proportion of ulcers healed after a 6 week course'. Treatments could be compared according to the cost per ulcer healed. However, if the relapse rates on the two drugs were very different, drug A might be falsely deemed 'more cost-effective' than drug B. A better outcome measure here might be 'ulcers which remained healed at 1 year'.

In cost–benefit analysis, where health status is expressed in utility units, such as QALYs, you would, if you were being really rigorous about evaluating the paper, look back at how the particular utilities used in the analysis were derived (see Section 10.2). In particular, you will want to know whose health preference values were used – those of patients, doctors, health economists or the government.

For a more detailed and surprisingly readable account of how to 'cost' different health care interventions, see the report from the UK Health Technology Assessment programme.[39]

Question 7: were incremental, rather than absolute, benefits considered?

This question is best illustrated by a simple example. Let's say drug X, at £100 per course, cures 10 out of every 20 patients. Its new competitor, drug Y, costs £120 per course and cures 11 out of 20 patients. The cost per case cured with drug X is £200 (since you spent £2000 curing 10 people), and the cost per case cured with drug Y is £218 (since you spent £2400 curing 11 people).

The *incremental* cost of drug Y – that is, the extra cost of curing the extra patient – is NOT £18 but £400, since this is the total amount extra that you have had to pay to achieve an outcome over and above what you would have achieved by giving all patients the cheaper drug. This striking example should be borne in mind the next time a pharmaceutical representative tries to persuade you that his or her product is 'more effective and only marginally more expensive'.

Question 8: was the 'here and now' given precedence over the distant future?

A bird in the hand is worth two in the bush. In health as well as money terms, we value a benefit today more highly than we value a promise of the same benefit in 5 years' time. When the costs or benefits of an intervention (or lack of the intervention) will occur some time in the future, their value should be *discounted* to reflect this. The actual amount of discount that should be allowed for future, as opposed to immediate, health benefit, is pretty arbitrary, but most analyses use a figure of around 5% per year.

Question 9: was a sensitivity analysis performed?

Let's say a cost–benefit analysis comes out as saying that hernia repair by day-case surgery costs £1500 per QALY whereas traditional open repair, with its associated hospital stay, costs £2100 per QALY. But, when you look at how the calculations were done, you are surprised at how cheaply the laparoscopic equipment has been costed. If you raise the price of this equipment by 25%, does day-case surgery still come out dramatically cheaper? It may, or it may not.

Sensitivity analysis, or exploration of 'what-ifs', was described in Section 8.2 in relation to meta-analysis. Exactly the same principles apply here: if adjusting the figures to account for the full range of possible influences gives you a totally different answer, you should not place too much reliance on the analysis. For a good example of a sensitivity analysis on a topic of both scientific and political importance, see Pharoah and Hollingworth's paper on the cost-effectiveness of lowering cholesterol (which addresses the difficult issue of who should receive, and who should be denied, effective but expensive cholesterol-lowering drugs).[40]

Question 10: were 'bottom line' aggregate scores overused?

In Section 10.2, I introduced the notion of cost–consequences analysis, in which the reader of the paper can attach his or her own values to different utilities. In practice, this is an unusual way of presenting an economic analysis, and, more commonly, the reader is faced with a cost–utility or cost–benefit analysis which gives a composite score in unfamiliar units which do not translate readily into exactly what gains and losses the patient can expect. The situation is analogous to the father who is told, 'your child's intelligence quotient is 115', when he would feel far better informed if he were presented with the disaggregated data: 'Johnny can read, write, count and draw pretty well for his age'.

10.4 Conclusion

I hope this chapter has shown that the critical appraisal of an economic analysis rests as crucially on asking questions such as, 'where did those numbers come from'? and 'have any numbers been left out'? as on checking that the sums themselves were correct. While few papers will fulfil all the criteria listed in Section 10.3 and summarised in Appendix 1, you should, after reading the chapter, be able to distinguish an economic analysis of moderate or good methodological quality from one which slips 'throwaway costings' ('drug X costs less than drug Y; therefore it is more cost-effective') into its results or discussion section.

References

1 Drummond MF, Jefferson TO. Guidelines for authors and peer reviewers of economic submissions to the BMJ. The BMJ Economic Evaluation Working Party. *BMJ* 1996;**313**:275–83.

2 O'Brien BJ, Heyland D, Richardson WS, Levine M, Drummond MF. Users' guides to the medical literature. XIII. How to use an article on economic analysis of clinical practice. B. What are the results and will they help me in caring for my patients? Evidence-Based Medicine Working Group [published erratum appears in *JAMA* 1997;**278**(13):1064]. *JAMA* 1997;**277**:1802–6.

3 Drummond MF, Richardson WS, O'Brien BJ, Levine M, Heyland D. Users' guides to the medical literature. XIII. How to use an article on economic analysis of clinical practice. A. Are the results of the study valid? Evidence-Based Medicine Working Group. *JAMA* 1997;277:1552–7.

4 Guyatt GH, Naylor CD, Juniper E, Heyland DK, Jaeschke R, Cook DJ. Users' guides to the medical literature. XII. How to use articles about health-related quality of life. Evidence-Based Medicine Working Group. *JAMA* 1997;277:1232–7.

5 Jefferson T, Demicheli V, Mugford M. *Elementary economic evaluation in health care*. London: BMJ Publications, 2000.

6 Klein R. The rationing debate. Defining a package in healthcare services the NHS is responsible for. The case against. *BMJ* 1997;314:506–9.

7 New B. The rationing debate. Defining a package of healthcare services the NHS is responsible for. The case for. *BMJ* 1997;314:503–5.

8 Culyer AJ. The rationing debate: maximising the health of the whole community. The case for. *BMJ* 1997;314:667–9.

9 Harris J. The rationing debate: maximising the health of the whole community. The case against: what the principal objective of the NHS should really be. *BMJ* 1997;314:669–72.

10 Williams A, Evans JG. The rationing debate. Rationing health care by age. *BMJ* 1997;314:820–5.

11 Lenaghan J. The rationing debate. Central government should have a greater role in rationing decisions. The case for. *BMJ* 1997;314:967–70.

12 Harrison S. The rationing debate. Central government should have a greater role in rationing decisions. The case against. *BMJ* 1997;314:970–3.

13 Doyal L. The rationing debate. Rationing within the NHS should be explicit. The case for. *BMJ* 1997;314:1114-18.

14 Coast J. The rationing debate. Rationing within the NHS should be explicit. The case against. *BMJ* 1997;314:1118–22.

15 Bowling A. *Measuring health*. Milton Keynes: Open University Press, 1997.

16 Bradley C. *Handbook of psychology and diabetes*. London: Psychology Press, 1986.

17 Bala MV, Wood LL, Zarkin GA, Norton EC, Gafni A, O'Brien B. Valuing outcomes in health care: a comparison of willingness to pay and quality-adjusted life-years. *J Clin Epidemiol* 1998;51:667–76.

18 Billingham LJ, Abrams KR, Jones DR. Methods for the analysis of quality-of-life and survival data in health technology assessment. *Health Technol Assess* 1999;3:1–152.

19 Birch S, Gafni A, Markham B, Marriott M, Lewis D, Main P. Health years equivalents as a measurement of preferences for dental interventions. *Community Dent Health* 1998;15:233–42.

20 Brazier J, Deverill M, Green C, Harper R, Booth A. A review of the use of health status measures in economic evaluation. *Health Technol Assess* 1999;3: i-164.

21 Brazier J, Roberts J, Deverill M. The estimation of a preference-based measure of health from the SF-36. *J Health Econ* 2002;21:271–92.

22 Fallowfield LJ, Harper P. Health-related quality of life in patients undergoing drug therapy for advanced non-small-cell lung cancer. *Lung Cancer* 2005;**48**:365–77.

23 Gafni A. Willingness-to-pay (WTP): the new-old kid on the economic evaluation block. *Can J Nurs Res* 2001;**33**:59–64.

24 Gill TM, Feinstein AR. A critical appraisal of the quality of quality-of-life measurements. *JAMA* 1994;**272**:619–26.

25 Guyatt GH, Cook DJ. Health status, quality of life, and the individual. *JAMA* 1994;**272**:630–1.

26 Macduff C. Respondent-generated quality of life measures: useful tools for nursing or more fool's gold? *J Adv Nurs* 2000;**32**:375–82.

27 Neudert C, Wasner M, Borasio GD. Patients' assessment of quality of life instruments: a randomised study of SIP, SF-36 and SEIQoL-DW in patients with amyotrophic lateral sclerosis. *J Neurol Sci* 2001;**191**:103–9.

28 Patel KK, Veenstra DL, Patrick DL. A review of selected patient-generated outcome measures and their application in clinical trials. *Value Health* 2003;**6**:595–603.

29 Brazier J, Deverill M, Green C. A review of the use of health status measures in economic evaluation. *J Health Serv Res Policy* 1999;**4**:174–84.

30 Hope T, Savulescu J, Hendrick J. Resource allocation. *Medical ethics and law; the core curriculum.* London: Churchill Livingstone, 2003.

31 Weinberger M, Oddone EZ, Samsa GP, Landsman PB. Are health-related quality-of-life measures affected by the mode of administration? *J Clin Epidemiol* 1996;**49**:135–40.

32 Harris J. QALYfying the value of life. *J Med Ethics* 1987;**13**:117–23.

33 Gafni A, Birch S. QALYs and HYEs (healthy years equivalent). Spotting the differences. *J Health Econ* 1997;**16**:601–8.

34 Birch S, Gafni A, O'Brien B. Willingness to pay and the valuation of programmes for the prevention and control of influenza. *Pharmacoeconomics* 1999;**16** (Suppl 1):55–61.

35 Gafni A. Willingness to pay in the context of an economic evaluation of healthcare programs: theory and practice. *Am J Manag Care* 1997;**3** (Suppl):S21–S32.

36 Gwatkin DR, Guillot M, Heuveline P. The burden of disease among the global poor. *Lancet* 1999;**354**:586–9.

37 Ustun TB, Rehm J, Chatterji S, Saxena S, Trotter R, Room R *et al.* Multiple-informant ranking of the disabling effects of different health conditions in 14 countries. WHO/NIH Joint Project CAR Study Group. *Lancet* 1999;**354**:111–15.

38 Arnesen T, Nord E. The value of DALY life: problems with ethics and validity of disability adjusted life years. *BMJ* 1999;**319**:1423–5.

39 Johnston K, Buxton MJ, Jones DR, Fitzpatrick R. Assessing the costs of healthcare technologies in clinical trials. *Health Technol Assess* 1999;**3**:1–76.

40 Pharoah PD, Hollingworth W. Cost effectiveness of lowering cholesterol concentration with statins in patients with and without pre-existing coronary heart disease: life table method applied to health authority population. *BMJ* 1996;**312**:1443–8.

Chapter 11 **Papers that go beyond numbers (qualitative research)**

11.1 What is qualitative research?

The pendulum is swinging. Twenty years ago, when I took up my first research post, a work-weary colleague advised me: 'Find something to measure, and keep on measuring it until you've got a boxful of data. Then stop measuring and start writing up'.

'But what should I measure'?, I asked.

'That', he said cynically, 'doesn't much matter'.

This true example illustrates the limitations of an exclusively quantitative (counting-and-measuring) perspective in research. Epidemiologist Nick Black has argued that a finding or a result is more likely to be accepted as a fact if it is quantified (expressed in numbers) than if it is not.[1] There is little or no scientific evidence, for example, to support the well-known 'facts' that 1 couple in 10 is infertile, 1 man in 10 is homosexual, and 1% of the children of first-cousin marriages have a genetic disorder. Yet, observes Black, most of us are happy to accept uncritically such simplified, reductionist and blatantly incorrect statements so long as they contain at least one number.

Qualitative researchers seek a deeper truth. They aim to 'study things in their natural setting, attempting to make sense of, or interpret, phenomena in terms of the meanings people bring to them',[2] and they use 'a holistic perspective which preserves the complexities of human behaviour'.[3]

Interpretive or qualitative research was for years the territory of social scientists. It is now increasingly recognised as being not just complementary to but, in many cases, a prerequisite for the quantitative research with which most us who trained in the biomedical sciences are more familiar. Certainly, the view that the two approaches are mutually exclusive has itself become 'unscientific', and it is currently rather trendy, particularly in the fields of primary care and health services research, to say that you are doing some qualitative research. Since the first edition of this book was published, qualitative research has even become mainstream within the evidence-based medicine movement,[3–5] and there have been major developments in the science of integrating qualitative and quantitative evidence in both individual clinical trials[6–8] and systematic review.[9]

Dr Cecil Helman, author of a leading textbook on the anthropological aspects of health and illness,[10] told me the following story to illustrate the qualitative–quantitative dichotomy.

A small child runs in from the garden and says, excitedly, 'Mummy, the leaves are falling off the trees'.

'Tell me more', says his mother.

'Well, five leaves fell in the first hour, then ten leaves fell in the second hour ...'

That child will become a quantitative researcher.

A second child, when asked 'tell me more', might reply, 'Well, the leaves are big and flat, and mostly yellow or red, and they seem to be falling off some trees but not others. And mummy, why did no leaves fall last month'?

That child will become a qualitative researcher.

Questions such as 'How many parents would consult their general practitioner when their child has a mild temperature'?, or 'What proportion of smokers have tried to give up'? clearly need answering through quantitative methods. But questions like 'Why do parents worry so much about their children's temperature'?, and 'What stops people from giving up smoking'? cannot and should not be answered by leaping in and measuring the first aspect of the problem that we (the outsiders) think might be important. Rather, we need to hang out, listen to what people have to say and explore the ideas and concerns which the subjects themselves come up with. After a while, we may notice a pattern emerging, which may prompt us to make our observations in a different way. We may start with one of the methods shown in Table 11.1, and go on to use a selection of others.

Box 11.1, which is reproduced with permission from Nick Mays and Catherine Pope's introductory book *Qualitative research in health care*[11] summarises (indeed overstates) the differences between the qualitative and quantitative approaches to research. In reality, there is a great deal of overlap between them, the importance of which is increasingly being recognised.[8,9]

As Section 3.2 explains, quantitative research should begin with an idea (usually articulated as a hypothesis), which then, through measurement, generates data and, by *deduction*, allows a conclusion to be drawn. Qualitative research is different. It begins with an intention to explore a particular area, collects 'data' (e.g. observations, interviews, documents – even emails can count as qualitative data), and generates ideas and hypotheses from these data largely through what is known as *inductive reasoning*.[2] The strength of quantitative approach lies in its *reliability* (repeatability) – that is, the same

Table 11.1 Examples of qualitative research methods

Documents	Study of documents produced by real people for real purposes, for example, minutes of meetings
Passive observation	Systematic watching of behaviour and talk in natural occurring settings
Participant-observation	Observation in which the researcher also occupies a role or part in the setting in addition to observing
Semi-structured interview	Face-to-face (or telephone) conversation with the purpose of exploring issues or topics in detail. Uses a broad list of questions or topics (known as a 'topic guide')
Narrative interview	Interview undertaken in a less structured fashion, with the purpose of getting a long story from the interviewee (typically a life story or the story of how an illness has unfolded over time). The interviewer holds back from prompting except to say 'tell me more'
Focus groups	Method of group interview which explicitly includes and uses the group interaction to generate data

Box 11.1 Qualitative versus quantitative research – the overstated dichotomy (see reference 11)

	Qualitative	Quantitative
Social theory	Action	Structure
Methods	Observation, interview	Experiment, survey
Question	What is X? (classification)	How many Xs? (enumeration)
Reasoning	Inductive	Deductive
Sampling method	Theoretical	Statistical
Strength	Validity	Reliability

Reproduced with permission from reference 11.

measurements should yield the same results time after time. The strength of qualitative research lies in *validity* (closeness to the truth) – that is, good qualitative research, using a selection of data collection methods, really should touch the core of what is going on rather than just skimming the surface. The validity of qualitative methods is greatly improved by the use of more than one method (see Table 11.1) in combination (a process sometimes known as *triangulation*), by the researcher thinking carefully about what is going on and how their own perspective might be influencing the data (an approach known as *reflexivity*),[12] and – some would argue – by more than one researcher analysing the same data independently (to demonstrate *inter-rater reliability*).

Since I wrote the first edition of this book, inter-rater reliability has become less credible as a measure of quality in qualitative research. Appraisers of qualitative papers increasingly seek to assess the competence and reflexivity of a single researcher rather than confirm that the findings were 'checked by someone else'. This change is attributable to two important insights. First, in most qualitative research, one person knows the data far better than anyone else, so the idea that two heads are better than one simply isn't true – a researcher who has been brought in merely to verify 'themes' may rely far more on personal preconceptions and guesswork than the main fieldworker. And second, with the trend towards more people from biomedical backgrounds doing qualitative research, it's not at all uncommon for two (or even a whole team of) naïve and untrained researchers setting up focus groups or attacking the free-text responses of questionnaires. Not only does 'agreement' between these individuals not correspond to quality, but teams from similar backgrounds are also likely to bring similar biases, so high inter-rater reliability scores may be entirely spurious.

Those who are ignorant about qualitative research often believe that it constitutes little more than hanging out and watching leaves fall. It is beyond the scope of this book to take you through the substantial literature on how to (and how not to) proceed when observing, interviewing, leading a focus group and so on. But sophisticated methods for all these techniques certainly exist, and if you are interested I suggest you try the introductory[13,14] or more detailed [2,15,16] texts listed at the end of this chapter.

Qualitative methods really come into their own when researching uncharted territory – that is, where the variables of greatest concern are poorly understood, ill-defined and cannot be controlled.[11] In such circumstances, the definitive hypothesis may not be arrived at until the study is well underway. But it is in precisely these circumstances that the qualitative researcher must ensure that (s)he has, at the outset, carefully delineated a particular focus of research and identified some specific questions to try to answer (see Question 1 in Section 11.2). The methods of qualitative research allow for – indeed, they require – modification of the research question in the light of findings generated along the way – a technique known as 'progressive focussing'.[11,16] (In contrast, as Section 5.2d showed, sneaking a look at the interim results of a quantitative study is statistically invalid!)

The so-called *iterative* approach (altering the research methods and the hypothesis as you go along) employed by qualitative researchers shows a commendable sensitivity to the richness and variability of the subject matter. Failure to recognise the legitimacy of this approach has, in the past, led critics to accuse qualitative researchers of continually moving their own goalposts. While these criticisms are often misguided, there is, as Nicky Britten and colleagues have observed, a real danger 'that the flexibility [of the iterative approach] will slide into sloppiness as the researcher ceases to be clear about what it is (s)he is investigating'.[17] They warn that qualitative researchers must, therefore, allow periods away from their fieldwork for reflection, planning and consultation with colleagues.

11.2 Evaluating papers that describe qualitative research

By its very nature, qualitative research is non-standard, unconfined and dependent on the subjective experience of both the researcher and the researched. It explores what needs to be explored and cuts its cloth accordingly. As implied in the previous section, qualitative research is an in-depth, interpretive task, not a technical procedure. It depends crucially on a competent and experienced researcher exercising the kind of skills and judgements that are difficult if not impossible to measure objectively. It is debatable, therefore, whether an all-encompassing critical appraisal checklist along the lines of the Users' Guides to the Medical Literature for quantitative research (see reference list for Chapter 3) could ever be developed, though attempts have been made.[4,5,18] Some people have argued that critical appraisal checklists potentially detract from research quality in qualitative research because they encourage a mechanistic and protocol-driven approach.[19,20]

My own view, and that of a number of individuals who have attempted, or are currently working on, this very task, is that such a checklist may not be as exhaustive or as universally applicable as the various guides for appraising quantitative research, but that it is certainly possible to set some ground rules. Without doubt, the best attempt to offer guidance (and also the best exposition of the uncertainties and unknowables) has been made by Mary Dixon-Woods and her colleagues.[21] The list which follows has been distilled from the published work cited elsewhere in this chapter, and also from discussions many years ago with Dr Rod Taylor, who produced one of the earliest critical appraisal guides for qualitative papers.

Question 1: did the paper describe an important clinical problem addressed via a clearly formulated question?

In Section 3.2, I explained that one of the first things you should look for in any research paper is a statement of why the research was done and what specific question it addressed. Qualitative papers are no exception to this rule: there is absolutely no scientific value in interviewing or observing people just for the sake of it. Papers which cannot define their topic of research more closely than 'we decided to interview 20 patients with epilepsy' inspire little confidence that the researchers really knew what they were studying or why.

You might be more inclined to read on if the paper stated in its introduction something like, 'Epilepsy is a common and potentially disabling condition, and up to 20% of patients do not remain fit-free on medication. Antiepileptic medication is known to have unpleasant side effects, and several studies have shown that a high proportion of patients do not take their tablets regularly. We therefore decided to explore patients' beliefs about epilepsy and their perceived reasons for not taking their medication'.

As I explained in Section 11.1, the iterative nature of qualitative research is such that the definitive research question may not be clearly focused at the outset of the study, but it should certainly have been formulated by the time the report is written!

Question 2: was a qualitative approach appropriate?

If the objective of the research was to explore, interpret or obtain a deeper understanding of a particular clinical issue, qualitative methods were almost certainly the most appropriate ones to use. If, however, the research aimed to achieve some other goal (such as determining the incidence of a disease or the frequency of an adverse drug reaction, testing a cause-and-effect hypothesis or showing that one drug has a better risk–benefit ratio than another), qualitative methods are clearly inappropriate! If you think a case-control, cohort study or randomised trial would have been better suited to the research question posed in the paper than the qualitative methods that were actually used, you might like to compare that question with the examples in Section 3.3 to confirm your hunch.

Question 3: how were (a) the setting and (b) the subjects selected?

Look back at Box 11.1 which contrasts the *statistical* sampling methods of quantitative research with the *theoretical* ones of qualitative research. Let me explain what this means. In the earlier chapters of this book, particularly Section 4.2, I emphasised the importance, in quantitative research, of ensuring that a truly random sample of participants is recruited. A random sample will ensure that the results reflect, on average, the condition of the population from which the sample was drawn.

In qualitative research, however, we are not interested in an 'on-average' view of a patient population. We want to gain an in-depth understanding of the experience of particular individuals or groups, and we should, therefore, deliberately seek out individuals or groups who fit the bill. If, for example, we wished to study the experience of women when they gave birth in hospital, we would be perfectly justified in going out of our way to find women who had had a range of different birth experiences – an induced delivery, an emergency Caesarean section, a delivery by a medical student, a late miscarriage and so on.

We would also wish to select some women who had shared antenatal care between an obstetrician and their general practitioner, and some women who had been cared for by community midwives throughout the pregnancy. In this example, it might be particularly instructive to find women who had had their care provided by male doctors, even though this would be a relatively unusual situation. Finally, we might choose to study patients who gave birth in the setting of a large, modern, 'high-tech' maternity unit as well as some who did so in a small community hospital. Of course, all these specifications will give us 'biased' samples, but that is exactly what we want.

Watch out for qualitative research where the sample has been selected (or appears to have been selected) purely on the basis of convenience. In the above example, taking the first dozen patients to pass through the nearest labour ward would be the easiest way to notch up interviews, but the information obtained may be considerably less helpful.

Question 4: what was the researcher's perspective, and has this been taken into account?

Given that qualitative research is necessarily grounded in real-life experience, a paper describing such research should not be 'trashed' simply because the researchers have declared a particular cultural perspective or personal involvement with the participants of the research. Quite the reverse: they should be congratulated for doing just that. It is important to recognise that there is no way of abolishing, or fully controlling for, observer bias in qualitative research. This is most obviously the case not only when participant observation (see Table 11.1) is used, but it is also true for other forms of data collection and data analysis.

If, for example, the research concerns the experience of adults with asthma living in damp and overcrowded housing and the perceived effect of these surroundings on their health, the data generated by techniques such as focus groups or semi-structured interviews are likely to be heavily influenced by what the *interviewer* believes about this subject and by whether he or she is employed by the hospital chest clinic, the social work department of the local authority or an environmental pressure group. But since it is inconceivable that the interviews could have been conducted by someone with no views at all and no ideological or cultural perspective, the most that can be required of the researchers is that they describe in detail where they are coming from so that the results can be interpreted accordingly.

It is for this reason, incidentally, that qualitative researchers generally prefer to write up their work in the first person ('I interviewed the participants' rather than 'the participants were interviewed'), because this makes explicit the role and influence of the researcher.

Question 5: what methods did the researcher use for collecting data – and are these described in enough detail?

I once spent two years doing highly quantitative, laboratory-based experimental research in which around 15 h of every week were spent filling or emptying test tubes. There was a standard way to fill the test tubes, a standard way to spin them in the centrifuge, and even a standard way to wash them up. When I finally published my research, some 900 h of drudgery was summed up in a single sentence: 'Patients' serum rhubarb levels were measured according to the method described by Bloggs and Bloggs [reference to Bloggs and Bloggs's paper on how to measure serum rhubarb]'.

I now spend quite a lot of my time doing qualitative research, and I can confirm that it's infinitely more fun. My research assistant and I have spent the last year devising a unique combination of techniques to measure the beliefs, hopes, fears and attitudes of diabetic patients from a particular minority ethnic group (British Bangladeshis). We had to develop, for example, a valid way of simultaneously translating and transcribing interviews which were conducted in Sylheti, a complex dialect of Bengali which has no written form. We found that patients' attitudes appear to be heavily influenced by the presence of certain of their relatives in the room, so we contrived to interview some patients in both the presence and the absence of these key relatives.

I could go on describing the methods we devised to address this particular research issue,[22] but I have probably made my point: the methods section of a qualitative paper often cannot be written in shorthand or dismissed by reference to someone else's research techniques. It may have to be lengthy and discursive since it is telling a unique story without which the results cannot be interpreted. As with the sampling strategy, there are no hard-and-fast rules about exactly what details should be included in this section of the paper. You should simply ask, 'have I been given enough information about the methods used'?, and, if you have, use your common sense to assess, 'are these methods sensible and adequate ways of addressing the research question'?

Question 6: what methods did the researcher use to analyse the data – and what quality control measures were implemented?

The data analysis section of a qualitative research paper is the opportunity for the researcher(s) to demonstrate the difference between sense and nonsense. Having amassed a thick pile of completed interview transcripts or field notes, the genuine qualitative researcher has hardly begun. It is simply not good enough to flick through the text looking for 'interesting quotes' which support a particular theory. The researcher must find a *systematic* way of analysing his or her data, and, in particular, must seek to detect and interpret items of data that appear to contradict or challenge the theories derived from the majority. One of the best short articles on qualitative data analysis was published by Cathy Pope in the *British Medical Journal* a few years ago – look it out if you're new to this field and want to know where to start.[13] If you want the definitive textbook on qualitative research, which describes multiple different approaches to analysis, try the marvellous tome edited by Denzin and Lincoln.[2]

By far the commonest way of analyzing the kind of qualitative data that is generally collected in biomedical research is *thematic analysis.* In this, the researchers go through printouts of free text, draw up a list of broad themes and allocate coding categories to each. For example, a 'theme' might be patients' knowledge about their illness and within this theme, codes might include 'transmissible causes', 'supernatural causes', 'causes due to own behaviour' and so on. Note that these codes do not correspond to a conventional biomedical taxonomy ('genetic', 'infectious', 'metabolic' and so on) because the point of the research is to explore the interviewees' taxonomy, whether the researcher agrees with it or not. Thematic analysis is often tackled by drawing up a matrix or framework with a new column for each theme and a new row for each 'case' (e.g. an interview transcript), and cutting and pasting relevant segments of text into each box.[23] Another type of thematic analysis is the constant comparative method – in which each new piece of data is compared with the emerging summary of all the previous items, allowing step-by-step refinement of an emerging theory.[24]

Quite commonly these days, qualitative data analysis is done with the help of a computer programme such as ATLAS-TI or NVIVO, which makes it much easier to handle large datasets. The statements made by all the interviewees on a particular topic can be compared with one another, and sophisticated comparisons can be made such as 'did people who made statement A also tend to make statement B'? But remember, a qualitative computer programme does not analyse the data by autopilot, any more than a quantitative programme like SPSS can tell the researcher which statistical test to apply in each case! While the sentence 'data were analysed using NVIVO' might appear impressive, the GIGO (garbage in, garbage out) rule often applies. Excellent qualitative data analysis can occur using the VLDRT (very large dining room table) method, in which print-outs of (say) interviews are marked up with felt pens and (say) the constant comparative method is undertaken manually instead of electronically.

It's often difficult when writing up qualitative research to demonstrate how quality control was achieved. As mentioned in the previous section, just because the data have been analysed by more than one researcher does not necessarily assure rigour. Indeed, researchers who never disagree on their subjective judgements (is a particular paragraph in a patient's account really evidence of 'anxiety' or 'disempowerment' or 'trust'?) are probably not thinking hard enough about their own interpretations. The essence of quality in such circumstances is more to do with the level of critical dialogue between the researchers, and in *how* disagreements were exposed and resolved. In analysing my own research data on the health beliefs of British Bangladeshis with diabetes,[22] for example, three of us looked in turn at a typed interview transcript and assigned codings to particular statements. We then compared our decisions and argued (sometimes heatedly) about our disagreements. Our analysis revealed differences in the interpretation of certain statements which we were unable to fully resolve. For example, we never reached agreement about what the term 'exercise' means in this ethnic group. This did not mean that one of us was 'wrong' but that there were *inherent* ambiguities in the data. Perhaps, for example, this sample of interviewees were themselves confused about what the term 'exercise' meant and the benefits it offered to people with diabetes.

Question 7: are the results credible, and if so, are they clinically important?

We obviously cannot assess the credibility of qualitative results via the precision and accuracy of measuring devices, nor their significance via confidence intervals and numbers needed to treat. The most important tool to determine whether the results are sensible and believable, and whether they matter in practice, is plain common sense.

One important aspect of the results section to check is whether the authors cite actual data. Claims such as 'general practitioners did not usually recognise the value of audit' would be infinitely more credible if one or two verbatim quotes from the interviewees were reproduced to illustrate them. The results should be independently and objectively verifiable (e.g. by including longer segments of text in an appendix or online resource), and all quotes and examples should be indexed so that they can be traced back to an identifiable interviewee and data source.

Question 8: what conclusions were drawn, and are they justified by the results?

A quantitative research paper, presented in standard IMRAD format (see Section 3.1), should clearly distinguish the study's results (usually a set of numbers) from the interpretation of those results. The reader should have no difficulty separating what the researchers *found* from what they think it *means*. In qualitative research, however, such a distinction is rarely possible, since the results are by definition an interpretation of the data.

It is therefore necessary, when assessing the validity of qualitative research, to ask whether the interpretation placed on the data accords with common sense and that the researcher's personal, professional and cultural perspective is made explicit so the reader can assess the 'lens' through which the researcher has undertaken the fieldwork, analysis and interpretation. This can be a difficult exercise because the language we use to describe things tends to impugn meanings and motives which the subjects themselves may not share. Compare, for example, the two statements, 'three women went to the well to get water' and 'three women met at the well and each was carrying a pitcher'.

It is becoming a cliché that the conclusions of qualitative studies, like those of all research, should be 'grounded in evidence' – that is, that they should flow from what the researchers found in the field. Mays and Pope suggest three useful questions for determining whether the conclusions of a qualitative study are valid:[11]

1 How well does this analysis explain why people behave in the way they do?
2 How comprehensible would this explanation be to a thoughtful participant in the setting?
3 How well does the explanation cohere with what we already know?

Question 9: are the findings of the study transferable to other settings?

One of the commonest criticisms of qualitative research is that the findings of any qualitative study pertain only to the limited setting in which they were obtained. In fact, this is not necessarily any truer of qualitative research than of quantitative research. Look back at the example of women's birth experiences that I described in Question 3. A convenience sample of the first dozen women to give birth would provide little more than the collected experiences of these 12 women. A *purposive* sample as described in Question 3 would extend the transferability of the findings to women having a wide range of birth experience. But by making iterative adjustments to the sampling frame as the research study unfolds, the researchers will be able to develop a theoretical sample and test new theories as they emerge. For example (and note, I'm making this example up), the researchers might find that better educated women seem to have more psychologically traumatic experiences than less well-educated women. This might lead to a new theory about women's expectations (the better educated the woman, the more she expects a 'perfect birth experience'), which would in turn lead to a change in the purposive sampling strategy (we now want to find extremes of maternal education), and so on. The more the research has been driven by this kind of progressive focusing and iterative data analysis, the more its findings are likely to be transferable beyond the sample itself.

11.3 Conclusion

Doctors have traditionally placed high value on number-based data, which may in reality be misleading, reductionist and irrelevant to the real issues. The increasing popularity of qualitative research in the biomedical sciences has arisen largely because quantitative methods provided either no answers, or the wrong answers, to important questions in both clinical care and service delivery. If you still feel that qualitative research is necessarily second-rate by virtue of being a 'soft' science, you should be aware that you are out of step with the evidence.

In 1993, Catherine Pope and Nicky Britten presented at a conference a paper entitled 'Barriers to qualitative methods in the medical mindset', in which they showed their collection of rejection letters from biomedical journals.[25] The letters revealed a striking ignorance of qualitative methodology on the part of reviewers. In other words, the people who had rejected the papers often appeared to be incapable of distinguishing good qualitative research from bad.

Somewhat ironically, poor-quality qualitative papers now appear regularly in some medical journals, who appear to have undergone an about-face in editorial policy since Pope and Britten's exposure of the 'medical mindset'. I hope, therefore, that the questions listed above, and the references below, will assist reviewers in both camps: those who continue to reject qualitative papers for the wrong reasons, and those who have climbed on the qualitative bandwagon and are now *accepting* such papers for the wrong reasons! Note, however, that the critical appraisal of qualitative research is a relatively underdeveloped science, and the questions posed in this chapter are still being refined.

References

1 Black N. Why we need qualitative research. *J Epidemiol Community Health* 1994;**48**:425–6.

2 Denzin M, Lincoln P, eds. *Handbook of qualitative research*, 3rd edn. London: Sage, 2005.

3 Green J, Britten N. Qualitative research and evidence based medicine. *BMJ* 1998;**316**:1230–2.

4 Giacomini MK, Cook DJ. Users' guides to the medical literature: XXIII. Qualitative research in health care B. What are the results and how do they help me care for my patients? Evidence-Based Medicine Working Group. *JAMA* 2000;**284**:478–82.

5 Giacomini MK, Cook DJ. Users' guides to the medical literature: XXIII. Qualitative research in health care A. Are the results of the study valid? Evidence-Based Medicine Working Group. *JAMA* 2000;**284**:357–62.

6 Hawe P, Shiell A, Riley T. Complex interventions: how 'out of control' can a randomised controlled trial be? *BMJ* 2004;**328**:1561–3.

7 Campbell M, Fitzpatrick R, Haines A, Kinmonth AL, Sandercock P, Spiegelhalter D *et al*. Framework for design and evaluation of complex interventions to improve health. *BMJ* 2000;**321**:694–6.

8 Abell P. Methodological achievements in sociology over the past few decades with specific reference to the interplay of qualitative and quantitative methods. In: Bryant C, Becker H, eds. *What has sociology achieved?* London: Macmillan Publishing, 1990.

9 Dixon-Woods M, Agarwal S, Young B, Jones D, Sutton A. *Integrative approaches to qualitative and quantitative evidence*. London: Health Development Agency, 2004.

10 Helman C. *Culture, health and illness*, 3rd edn. London: Churchill Livingstone, 2004.

11 Mays N, Pope C. *Qualitative research in health care*, 2nd edn. London: BMJ Publications, 1999.

12 Koch T, Harrington A. Reconceptualizing rigour: the case for reflexivity. *J Adv Nurs* 1998;**28**:882–90.

13 Pope C, Ziebland S, Mays N. Qualitative research in health care. Analysing qualitative data. *BMJ* 2000;**320**:114–16.

14 Mays N, Pope C. Qualitative research in health care. Assessing quality in qualitative research. *BMJ* 2000;**320**:50–2.

15 Murphy E, Dingwall R, Greatbatch D, Parker S, Watson P. Qualitative research methods in health technology assessment: a review of the literature. *Health Technol Assess* 1998;**2**:50–2.

16 Silverman D. *Doing qualitative research – a practical handbook*. London: Sage, 1990.

17 Britten N, Jones R, Murphy E, Stacy R. Qualitative research methods in general practice and primary care. *Fam Pract* 1995;**12**:104–14.

18 Horsburgh D. Evaluation of qualitative research. *J Clin Nurs* 2003;**12**:307–12.

19 Sale JE, Hawker GA. Critical appraisal of qualitative research in clinical journals challenged. *Arthritis Rheum* 2005;**53**:314–16.

20 Barbour RS. Checklists for improving rigour in qualitative research: a case of the tail wagging the dog? *BMJ* 2001;**322**:1115–17.

21 Dixon-Woods M, Shaw RL, Agarwal S, Smith JA. The problem of appraising qualitative research. *Qual Saf Health Care* 2004;**13**:223–5.

22 Greenhalgh T, Helman C, Chowdhury AM. Health beliefs and folk models of diabetes in British Bangladeshis: a qualitative study. *BMJ* 1998;**316**:978–83.

23 Spencer L, Ritchie J, Lewis J, Dillon L. *Quality in qualitative evaluation: a framework for assessing research evidence.* London: Cabinet Office, 2003.

24 Glaser BG, Strauss AL. The constant comparative method of qualitative analysis. In: Glaser B, Strauss AL, eds. *The discovery of grounded theory.* Chicago: Adline, 1967.

25 Pope C, Britten N. The quality of rejection: barriers to qualitative methods in the medical mindset. *Paper presented at BSA Medical Sociology Group annual conference, September* 1993.

Chapter 12 **Papers that report questionnaire research**

12.1 The rise and rise of questionnaire research

When and where did you last fill out a questionnaire? They come through the door and appear in our pigeonholes at work. We get them as email attachments and find them in the dentist's waiting room. The kids bring them home from school, and it's not uncommon for one to accompany the bill in a restaurant. I recently met someone at a party who described himself as a 'questionnaire mugger' – his job was to stop people in the street and take down their answers to a list of questions about their income, tastes, shopping preferences and goodness knows what else.

This chapter, new for the third edition, is based on a series of papers I edited for the *British Medical Journal*, written by a team led by my lecturer Petra Boynton. [1–3] Petra has taught me lots about this widely used research technique, including the fact that there's probably more bad questionnaire research in the literature than just about any other category. Whereas you need a laboratory to do bad lab work, and a supply of medicines to do bad pharmaceutical research, all you need to do to produce bad questionnaire research is write out a list of questions, photocopy it and ask a few people to fill it in. It's therefore somewhat odd that the otherwise very comprehensive Users' Guides to the Medical Literature (see the reference list at the end of Chapter 3) do not include one on questionnaire studies.

Questionnaires are frequently touted as an 'objective' means of collecting information about people's knowledge, beliefs, attitudes and behaviour.[4,5] Do our patients like our opening hours? What do teenagers think of a local antidrugs campaign – and has it changed their attitudes? How much do nurses know about the management of asthma? What proportion of the population view themselves as gay or bisexual? Why don't doctors use computers to their maximum potential? You can probably see from these examples that questionnaires can seek both quantitative data (x percent of people like our services) and qualitative data (people using our services have xyz experiences). In other words, questionnaires are not a 'quantitative method' or a 'qualitative method' but a tool for collecting a range of different types of data, depending on the question asked in each item.

I've already used the expression GIGO (garbage in, garbage out) in previous chapters to make the point that poorly structured instruments lead to poor quality data, misleading conclusions and woolly recommendations. Nowhere is that more true than in questionnaire research. Whereas clear guidance on the design and reporting of randomized controlled trials is now widely available (see the discussion about the CONSORT checklist in Chapter 6), there is no comparable framework for questionnaire research. Perhaps for this reason, despite a wealth of detailed guidance in the specialist literature,[4] elementary methodological errors are common in questionnaire research undertaken by health professionals.[1–3]

Before we turn to the critical appraisal, a word about terminology. A questionnaire is a form of psychometric instrument – that is, it is designed to measure formally an aspect of human psychology. We sometimes refer to questionnaires as 'instruments'. The questions within a questionnaire are sometimes known as 'items'. An item is the smallest unit within the questionnaire that is individually scored. It might comprise a stem ('pick which of the following responses corresponds to your own view') and then five possible options. Or it might be a simple 'yes/no' or 'true/false' response.

12.2 Ten questions to ask about a paper describing a questionnaire study

Question 1: what was the research question, was the questionnaire appropriate for answering it?

Look back to Section 3.1, where I describe three preliminary questions to get you started in appraising any paper. The first of these was 'what was the research question – and why was the study needed?' This is a particularly good starter question for questionnaire studies, since (as explained in the previous section) inexperienced researchers often embark on questionnaire research without clarifying why they are doing it or what they want to find out. In addition, people often decide to use a questionnaire for studies that need a totally different method. Sometimes, a questionnaire will be appropriate but only if used within a mixed methodology study (e.g. to extend and quantify the findings of an initial exploratory phase). Table 12.1 gives some real examples based on papers that Petra Boynton and I collected from the published literature and offered by participants in courses we have run.

There are many advantages to researchers of using a previously validated and published questionnaire. The research team will save time and resources;

Table 12.1 Examples of research questions for which a questionnaire may *not* be the most appropriate design

Broad of area research	Example of research questions	Why is a questionnaire *not* the most appropriate method?	What method(s) should be used instead?
Burden of disease	What is the prevalence of asthma in school children?	A child may have asthma but the parent does not know it; parents may think incorrectly that their child has asthma; or they may withhold information that is perceived as stigmatizing	Cross-sectional survey using standardised diagnostic criteria and/or systematic analysis of medical records
Professional behaviour	How do general practitioners manage low back pain?	What doctors say they do is not the same as what they actually do, especially when they think their practice is being judged by others.	Direct observation or video recording of consultations; use of simulated patients; systematic analysis of medical records
Health-related lifestyle	What proportion of people in smoking cessation studies quit successfully?	The proportion of true quitters is less than the proportion who say they have quit. A similar pattern is seen in studies of dietary choices, exercise and other lifestyle factors	'Gold standard' diagnostic test (in this example, urinary or salivary cotinine)
Needs assess-ment in 'special needs' groups	What are the unmet needs of refugees and asylum seekers for health and social care services?	A questionnaire is likely to reflect the preconceptions of researchers (e.g. it may take existing services and/or the needs of more 'visible' groups as its starting point), and fail to tap into important areas of need	Range of exploratory qualitative methods designed to build up a 'rich picture' of the problem – for example, semi-structured interviews of users, health professionals and the voluntary sector; focus groups and in-depth studies of critical events

they will be able to compare their own findings with those from other studies; they need only give outline details of the instrument when they write up their work; and they will not need to have gone through a thorough validation process for the instrument. Sadly, inexperienced researchers (most typically, students doing a dissertation) tend to forget to look thoroughly in the literature for a suitable 'off the peg' instrument, and such individuals often don't know about formal validation techniques (see below). Even though most such studies will be rejected by journal editors, a worrying proportion find their way into the literature.

Increasingly, health services research uses standard 'off the peg' questionnaires designed explicitly for producing data that can be compared across studies. For example, clinical trials routinely include standard instruments to measure patients' knowledge about a disease,[6] satisfaction with services [7] or health-related quality of life (QoL).[8] The validity (see below) of this approach depends crucially on whether the type and range of closed responses (i.e. the list of possible answers that people are asked to select from) reflects the full range of perceptions and feelings that people in all the different potential sampling frames might actually hold.

Question 2: was the questionnaire used in the study valid and reliable?

A valid questionnaire measures what it claims to measure. In reality, many fail to do this. For example, a self-completion questionnaire that seeks to measure people's food intake may be invalid, since in reality it measures what they *say* they have eaten, not what they have *actually* eaten. [9] Similarly, questionnaires asking GPs how they manage particular clinical conditions have been shown to differ significantly from actual clinical practice. [10] Note that an instrument developed in a different time, country or cultural context may not be a valid measure in the group you are studying. Here's a quirky example. The item 'I often attend gay parties' was a valid measure of a person's sociability level in the United Kingdom in the 1950s, but the wording has a very different connotation today! If you're interested in the measurement of quality of life through questionnaires, you might like to look out the controversy about the validity of such instruments when used beyond the context in which they were developed.[11–16]

Reliable questionnaires yield consistent results from repeated samples and different researchers over time.[4] Differences in the results obtained from a reliable questionnaire come from differences between participants, and not from inconsistencies in how the items are understood or how different observers interpret the responses. A standardised questionnaire is one that is written and administered in a strictly set manner, so all participants are asked precisely the same questions in an identical format and responses are recorded in a uniform manner. Standardising a measure increases its reliability. If you participated in the United Kingdom Census (General Household Survey) in 2001, you may remember being asked a rather mechanical set of questions.

This is because the interviewer had been trained to administer the instrument in a highly standardized way, so as to increase reliability. It's often difficult to ascertain from a published paper how hard the researchers tried to achieve standardization, but they may have quoted inter-rater reliability figures.

Question 3: what did the questionnaire look like, and was this appropriate for the target population?

When I say 'what did it look like'? I'm talking about two things – form and content. Form concerns issues such as how many pages was it, was it visually appealing (or off-putting), how long did it take to fill in, the terminology used and so on. These are not minor issues! A questionnaire that goes on for 30 pages, includes reams of scientific jargon and contains questions that a respondent might find offensive will not be properly filled in – and hence the results of a survey will be meaningless.

Content is about the actual items. Did the questions make sense, and could the participants in the sample understand them? Were any questions ambiguous or overly complicated? Were ambiguous weasel words such as 'frequently', 'regularly', 'commonly', 'usually', 'many', 'some' and 'hardly ever' avoided? Were the items 'open' (respondents can write anything they like) or 'closed' (respondents must pick from a list of options) – and if the latter, were all potential responses represented? Closed-ended designs enable researchers to produce aggregated data quickly, but the range of possible answers is set by the researchers, not the respondents, and the richness of responses is therefore much lower.[17] Some respondents (known as 'yea-sayers') tend to agree with statements rather than disagree. For this reason, researchers should not present their items so that 'strongly agree' always links to the same broad attitude. For example, on a patient satisfaction scale, if one question is 'my GP generally tries to help me out', another question should be phrased in the negative – for example, 'the receptionists are usually *impolite*'.

Question 4: were the instructions clear?

If you have ever been asked to fill out a questionnaire and 'got lost' halfway through (or discovered you don't know where to send it once you've filled it in), you will know that instructions contribute crucially to the validity of the instrument. These include

1 an explanation of what the study is about and what the overall purpose of the research is;
2 an assurance of anonymity and confidentiality, as well as confirmation that the person can stop completing the questionnaire at any time without having to give a reason;

3 clear and accurate contact details of whom to approach for further information;
4 if a postal questionnaire, instructions on what they need to send back and a stamped addressed envelope;
5 adequate instructions on how to complete each item, with examples where necessary?
6 any insert (e.g. leaflet), gift (e.g. book token) or honorarium, if these are part of the protocol.

These aspects of the study are unlikely to be listed in the published paper, but they may be in an appendix, and if not, you should be able to get the information from the authors.

Question 5: was the questionnaire adequately piloted?

Questionnaires often fail because participants don't understand them, can't complete them, get bored or offended by them or dislike how they look. Although friends and colleagues can help check spelling, grammar and layout, they cannot reliably predict the emotional reactions or comprehension difficulties of other groups. For this reason, all questionnaires (whether newly developed or 'off the peg') should be piloted on participants who are representative of the definitive study sample to see, for example, how long people take to complete the instrument, whether any items are misunderstood, or whether people get bored or confused halfway through. Three specific questions to ask are (a) What were the characteristics of the participants on whom the instrument was piloted; (b) *How* was the piloting exercise undertaken – what details are given? and (c) *In what ways* was the definitive instrument changed as a result of piloting?

Question 6: what was the sample?

If you have read the previous chapters, you will know that a skewed or non-representative sample will lead to misleading results and unsafe conclusions. When you appraise a questionnaire study, it's important to ask what the sampling frame was for the definitive study (purposive, random, snowball) and also whether it was sufficiently large and representative (Table 12.2). The main types of sample for a questionnaire study are

1 *Random sample.* A target group is identified, and a random selection of people from that group is invited to participate. For example, a computer might be used to select a random one in four samples from a diabetes register.
2 *Stratified random sample.* As random sample but the target group is first stratified according to a particular characteristic(s) – for example, diabetic

Table 12.2 Types of sampling frame for questionnaire research

Sample type	How it works	When to use
Opportunity/haphazard	Participants are selected from a group who are available at the time of study (e.g. patients attending a GP surgery on a particular morning)	Should be avoided if possible
Random	A target group is identified, and a random selection of people from this group is invited to participate. For example, a computer might be used to select a random one in four sample from a diabetes register	Use in studies where you wish to reflect the average viewpoint of a population
Stratified random	As random sample but the target group is first stratified according to a particular characteristic(s) – for example, diabetic people on insulin, tablets and diet. Random sampling is done separately for these different subgroups	Use when the target group is likely to have systematic differences by subgroup
Quota	Participants who match the wider population are identified (e.g. into groups such as social class, gender age etc.). Researchers are given a set number within each group to interview (e.g. so many young middle-class women)	For studies where you want to reflect outcomes as closely representative of the wider population as possible. Frequently used in political opinion polls etc.
Snowball	Participants are recruited and asked to identify other similar people to take part in the research	Helpful when working with hard-to-reach groups (e.g. lesbian mothers)

people on insulin, tablets and diet. Random sampling is done separately for these different subgroups.

3 *Snowball sample.* A small group of participants is identified and then asked to 'invite a friend' to complete the questionnaire. This group is in turn invited to nominate someone else, and so on.

4 *Opportunity.* Usually for pragmatic reasons, the first people to appear who meet the criteria are asked to complete the questionnaire. This might happen, for example, in a busy GP surgery when all patients attending on a particular day are asked to fill out a survey about the convenience of opening hours. But such a sample is clearly biased, since those who find the opening hours inconvenient won't be there in the first place! This example should remind you that opportunity (sometimes known as convenience) samples are rarely if ever scientifically justified.

It is also important to consider whether the instrument was suitable for all participants and potential participants. In particular, did it take account of the likely range in the sample of physical and intellectual abilities, language and literacy, understanding of numbers or scaling, and perceived threat of questions or questioner?

Question 7: how was the questionnaire administered – and was the response rate adequate?

The methods section of a paper describing a questionnaire study should include details of three aspects of administration: (a) How was the questionnaire distributed (e.g. by post, face to face or electronically)? (b) How was the questionnaire completed (e.g. self-completion or researcher-assisted)? and (c) Were the response rates reported fully, including details of participants who were unsuitable for the research or refused to take part? Have any potential response biases been discussed?

The *British Medical Journal* will not usually publish a paper if fewer than 70% of people approached completed the questionnaire properly. There have been a number of research studies on how to increase the response rate to a questionnaire study. In summary, the following have all been shown to increase response rates: [1,4,5]

• The questionnaire is clearly designed and has a simple layout
• It offers participants incentives or prizes in return for completion
• It has been thoroughly piloted and tested
• Participants are notified about the study in advance, with a personalised invitation
• The aim of study and means of completing the questionnaire are clearly explained

- A researcher is on-hand to answer questions and collect the completed questionnaire
- If using a postal questionnaire, a stamped addressed envelope is included
- The participant feels he or she is a stakeholder in the study
- Questions are phrased in a way that holds the participant's attention
- The questionnaire has clear focus and purpose, and is kept concise
- The questionnaire is appealing to look at.

Another thing to look for in relation to response rates is a table in the paper comparing the characteristics of people who responded with people who were approached but refused to fill out the questionnaire. If there were systematic (as opposed to chance) differences between these groups, the results of the survey will not be generalisable to the population from which the responders were drawn. Responders to surveys conducted in the street, for example, are often older than average (perhaps because they're in less of a hurry!), and less likely to be from an ethnic minority (perhaps because some ethnic individuals are unable to speak English fluently). On the other hand, if the authors of the study have shown that non-responders are pretty similar to responders, you should worry less about generalisability even if response rates were lower than you'd have liked.

Question 8: how were the data analysed?
Analysis of questionnaire data is a sophisticated science. See Oppenheim's excellent textbook if you're interested in learning the formal techniques.[4] If you're just interested in completing a checklist about a published question-naire study, try considering these aspects of the study. First, broadly what sort of analysis was carried out and was this appropriate? In particular, were the correct statistical tests used for quantitative responses,[4] and/or was a recog-nizable method of qualitative analysis (see Section 11.2) used for open-ended questions? It's reassuring (but by no means a flawless test) to learn that one of the paper's authors is a statistician. And as I said in Chapter 5, if the statistical tests used are ones you've never heard of, you should smell a rat. The vast majority of questionnaire data can be analysed using commonly used stat-istical tests such as Chi squared, Spearman's, Pearson correlation and so on. The commonest mistake of all in questionnaire research is to use no statistical tests at all, and you don't need a PhD in statistics to spot that dodge!

You should also check to ensure that there is no evidence of 'data dredging'. In other words, have the authors simply thrown their data into a computer and run hundreds of tests, and then dreamt up a plausible hypothesis to go with something that comes out as 'significant?' In the jargon, all analyses should be hypothesis driven – that is, the hypothesis should be thought up first and then the analysis should be done, not vice versa.

Question 9: what were the main results?

Consider first what the overall results were, and whether all relevant data were reported. Are quantitative results definitive (statistically significant) and are relevant non-significant results also reported? Have qualitative results been adequately interpreted (e.g. using an explicit theoretical framework), and have any quotes been properly justified and contextualized (rather than 'cherry picked' to spice up the paper)? Look back at Chapter 6 ('Papers that report drug trials') and remind yourself of the tricks used by unscrupulous marketing people to oversell findings. Check carefully the graphs (especially the zero-intercept on axes) and the data tables.

Question 10: what are the key conclusions?

This is a common sense question. What do the results actually mean, and have the researchers drawn an appropriate link between the data and their conclusions? Have the findings been placed within the wider body of knowledge in the field (especially any similar or contrasting surveys using the same instrument)? Have the authors acknowledged the limitations of their study and couched their discussion in the light of these (e.g. if the sample was small or the response rate low, did they recommend further studies to confirm the preliminary findings)? Finally, are any recommendations fully justified by the findings? For example, if they have done a small, parochial study they should not be suggesting changes in national policy as a result!

In conclusion, anyone can write down a list of questions and photocopy it – but this doesn't mean that a set of responses to these questions constitutes research! The development, administration, analysis and reporting of questionnaire studies is at least as challenging as the other research approaches described in other chapters in this book. In future editions, I hope to be able to refer to a structured reporting format comparable to CONSORT (RCTs), QUORUM (systematic reviews) and AGREE (guidelines), and I suspect that once such a format has been around for a few years, papers describing questionnaire research will be more consistent and easier to appraise.

References

1 Boynton PM. A hands on guide to questionnaire research part two: administering, analysing, and reporting your questionnaire. *BMJ* 2004;**328**:1372–5.

2 Boynton PM, Greenhalgh T. A hands on guide to questionnaire research part one: selecting, designing, and developing your questionnaire. *BMJ* 2004;**328**:1312–15.

3 Boynton PM, Wood GW, Greenhalgh T. A hands on guide to questionnaire research part three: reaching beyond the white middle classes. *BMJ* 2004;**328**:1433–6.

4 Oppenheim AN. *Questionnaire design, interviewing and attitude measurement.* London and New York: Continuum, 1992.

5 Sapsford R. *Survey research.* London and New Delhi: Sage and Thousand Oaks, 1999.

6 Bradley C. *Handbook of psychology and diabetes.* London: Psychology Press, 1986.

7 Howie JG, Heaney DJ, Maxwell M, Walker JJ. A comparison of a Patient Enablement Instrument (PEI) against two established satisfaction scales as an outcome measure of primary care consultations. *Fam Pract* 1998;**15**:165–71.

8 Billingham LJ, Abrams KR, Jones DR. Methods for the analysis of quality-of-life and survival data in health technology assessment. *Health Technol Assess* 1999;**3**:1–152.

9 Drewnowski A. Diet image: a new perspective on the food-frequency questionnaire. *Nutr Rev* 2001;**59**:370–2.

10 Adams AS, Soumerai SB, Lomas J, Ross-Degnan D. Evidence of self-report bias in assessing adherence to guidelines. *Int J Qual Health Care* 1999;**11**:187–92.

11 Scientific Advisory Committee of the Medical Outcomes Trust. Assessing health status and quality-of-life instruments: attributes and review criteria. *Qual Life Res* 2002;**11**:193–205.

12 Anderson RT, Aaronson NK, Bullinger M, McBee WL. A review of the progress towards developing health-related quality-of-life instruments for international clinical studies and outcomes research. *Pharmacoeconomics* 1996;**10**:336–55.

13 Beurskens AJ, de Vet HC, Koke AJ, van der Heijden GJ, Knipschild PG. Measuring the functional status of patients with low back pain. Assessment of the quality of four disease-specific questionnaires. *Spine* 1995;**20**:1017–28.

14 Bouchard S, Pelletier MH, Gauthier JG, Cote G, Laberge B. The assessment of panic using self-report: a comprehensive survey of validated instruments. *J Anxiety Disord* 1997;**11**:89–111.

15 Dijkers M. Measuring quality of life: methodological issues. *Am J Phys Med Rehabil* 1999;**78**:286–300.

16 Gilbody SM, House AO, Sheldon T. Routine administration of Health Related Quality of Life (HRQoL) and needs assessment instruments to improve psychological outcome – a systematic review. *Psychol Med* 2002;**32**:1345–56.

17 Houtkoop-Steenstra H. *Interaction and the standardized survey interview: the living questionnaire.* Cambridge: Cambridge University Press, 2000.

Chapter 13 **Getting evidence into practice**

13.1 Why are health professionals slow to adopt evidence-based practice?

Health professionals' failure to practice in accordance with the best available evidence cannot be attributed entirely to ignorance or stubbornness. Consultant paediatrician Dr Vivienne Van Someren has described an example that illustrates many of the additional barriers to getting research evidence into practice: the prevention of neonatal respiratory distress syndrome in premature babies.[1]

It was discovered back in 1957 that babies born more than 6 weeks early may get into severe breathing difficulties because of lack of a substance called surfactant, which lowers the surface tension within the lung alveoli and reduces resistance to expansion. Pharmaceutical companies began research in the 1960s to develop an artificial surfactant that could be given to the infant to prevent the life-threatening syndrome developing, but it was not until the mid-1980s that an effective product was developed.

By the late 1980s a number of randomised trials had taken place, and a meta-analysis published in 1990 suggested that the benefits of artificial surfactant greatly outweighed its risks. In 1990, a 6000-patient trial (OSIRIS) was begun which involved almost all the major neonatal intensive care units in the United Kingdom. The manufacturer was awarded a product licence in 1990, and by 1993, practically every eligible premature infant in the United Kingdom was receiving artificial surfactant.

Another treatment had also been shown a generation earlier to prevent neonatal respiratory distress syndrome: administration of the steroid drug dexamethasone to mothers in premature labour. Dexamethasone worked by accelerating the rate at which the fetal lung reached maturity. Its efficacy had been demonstrated in experimental animals in 1969, and in clinical trials on humans, published in the prestigious journal *Paediatrics*, as early as 1972. Yet despite a significant beneficial effect being confirmed in a number of further trials, and a meta-analysis published in 1990, the take-up of this technology

Table 13.1 Factors influencing implementation of evidence to prevent neonatal respiratory distress syndrome (Dr V Van Someren, personal communication)

	Surfactant treatment	Prenatal steroid treatment
Perception of mechanism	Corrects a surfactant deficiency disease	Ill-defined effect on developing lung tissue
Timing of effect	Minutes	Days
Impact on prescriber	Views effect directly (has to stand by ventilator)	Sees effect as statistic in annual report
Perception of side effects	Perceived as minimal	Clinicians' and patients' anxiety disproportionate to actual risk
Conflict between two patients	No (paediatrician's patient will benefit directly)	Yes (obstetrician's patient will not benefit directly)
Pharmaceutical industry interest	High (patented product; huge potential revenue)	Low (product out of patent; small potential revenue)
Trial technology	'New' (developed in late 1980s)	'Old' (developed in early 1970s)
Widespread involvement of clinicians in trials	Yes	No

was astonishingly slow. It was estimated in 1995 that only 12–18% of eligible mothers currently received this treatment in the United States.[2]

The quality of the evidence and the magnitude of the effect were similar for both these interventions.[3,4] Why were the paediatricians so much quicker than the obstetricians at implementing an intervention which prevented avoidable deaths? Dr Van Someren has considered a number of factors, listed in Table 13.1.[1] The effect of artificial surfactant is virtually immediate, and the doctor administering it witnesses directly the 'cure' of a terminally sick baby. Pharmaceutical industry support for a large (and, arguably, scientifically unnecessary) trial ensured that few consultant paediatricians appointed in the early 1990s would have escaped being introduced to the new technology.

In contrast, steroids, particularly for pregnant women, were unfashionable and perceived by patients to be 'bad for you'. In doctors' eyes, dexamethasone was an old hat treatment for a host of unglamorous diseases, notably end-stage cancer, and the scientific mechanism for its effect on fetal lungs was not readily understood. Most poignantly of all, an obstetrician would rarely get a chance to witness directly the life-saving effect on an individual patient.

The above example is far from isolated. Effective health care strategies frequently (though thankfully not always) take years to catch on, even amongst the experts who should be at the cutting edge of practice.[5–8] The remaining sections in this chapter consider how we can reduce the time from research evidence appearing to making real differences in health outcomes. And be warned – there are no quick fixes.

13.2 How can we influence health professionals' behaviour to promote evidence-based practice?

The Cochrane Effective Practice and Organisation of Care Group (EPOC, described in Chapter 9, p.141) have done an excellent job of summarising the literature accumulated from research trials on what is and is not effective in changing professional practice – both in promoting effective innovations and in encouraging professionals to resist 'innovations' that are ineffective or harmful.[9] EPOC have been mainly interested in reviewing trials of interventions aimed at redressing potential gaps in the evidence-into-practice sequence.

One of the few unequivocal messages from EPOC's work is that simply *telling* people about evidence-based medicine is consistently ineffective at changing practice. Until relatively recently, education (at least in relation to the training of doctors) was more or less synonymous with the didactic talk-and-chalk sessions that most of us remember from school and college. The 'bums on seats' approach to postgraduate education (filling lecture theatres up with doctors or nurses and wheeling on an 'expert' to impart pearls of wisdom) is relatively cheap and convenient for the educators but does not lead to sustained behaviour change in practice.[10–12] Indeed, one study demonstrated that the number of reported 'CME' (continuing medical education) hours attended was *inversely* correlated with doctors' competence![13]

If, like me, you're interested in the theory underpinning EBM teaching, you will have spotted that the 'instructional' approach to promoting professional behaviour change in relation to EBM is built on the flawed assumption that people behave in a particular way *because (and only because) they lack knowledge*, and that imparting knowledge will therefore change behaviour. Theresa Marteau and colleagues' short and authoritative critique shows that this model has neither theoretical coherence nor empirical support.[14] Information, they conclude, may be *necessary* for professional behaviour change, but it is rarely if ever *sufficient*. Psychological theories that Marteau and her team felt might inform the design of more effective educational strategies include

1 Behavioural learning – the notion that behaviour is more likely to be repeated if it is associated with rewards, and less likely if it is punished;

2 Social cognition – when planning an action, individuals ask themselves 'Is it worth the cost'?, 'What do other people think about this'? and 'Am I capable of achieving it'?; and

3 Stages of change models – in which all individuals are considered to lie somewhere on a continuum of readiness to change from no awareness that there is a need to change through to sustained implementation of the desired behaviour.

So, what sort of educational approaches have actually been shown to be effective for promoting evidence-based practice? Here's a summary of the empirical literature, based mainly on three systematic reviews of intervention trials:[15–17]

1 EBM teaching as conventionally delivered in undergraduate medical education curricula improves students' EBM knowledge and attitudes, but an impact on their performance in dealing with real cases has not been convincingly demonstrated.

2 In relation to qualified doctors, most classroom-based EBM training has little or no impact on their knowledge or critical appraisal skills. This may be because both the training and the tests are non-compulsory, or it may be because the training itself is too little, too superficial, too formulaic, too passive and too removed from practice.[18]

3 More educationally sound approaches such as 'integrated' EBM teaching (e.g. during ward rounds or in the emergency room) [19] or intensive short courses using highly interactive learning methods [20] can produce significant changes in knowledge, skills and behaviour.

4 However, no direct impact has yet been demonstrated from such courses on any patient-relevant outcomes.[18,21,22]

Michael Green, who has conducted one of the most rigorous primary studies of EBM training, as well as a national survey of programmes and a critical overview, [23–25] holds the view that EBM teaching should occur 'where the rubber meets the road' – that is, in the clinic and at the bedside.[25] He cites adult learning theory to support the argument that EBM teaching must surely be more effective if the learner can relate it to practical problems in the here-and-now and use it for real (as opposed to hypothetical) decision making. The way forward, he claims, is for more senior clinicians to follow Sackett's example and take an 'evidence cart' or equivalent on their rounds,[26] enabling clinical questions to be raised and answered in a context that optimises active learning.[25] For a useful article on theory-driven approaches to professional behaviour change, see Eccles and colleagues' review.[27]

In Chapter 9, I described the main findings of Jeremy Grimshaw's 2004 systematic review on guideline implementation.[28] The main conclusion of that review was that despite hundreds of studies costing millions of dollars, no intervention, either educational or otherwise, and either singly or in combination, is *guaranteed* to change the behaviour of practitioners in an 'evidence-based' direction. This conclusion is remarkably similar to that drawn by Andy Oxman's team in the famous 'No magic bullets' systematic review published in 1995 [12] and Richard Grol's narrative overview of 25 years' implementation research published in 1997.[29]

Here's where I part company slightly with the EPOC approach. Whereas many EPOC members are still undertaking trials (and reviews of trials) to add to the research base on whether this or that intervention (such leaflets and other printed educational materials, [30] audit and feedback [31] or financial incentives [32]) is or is not effective in changing clinician behaviour, my own view is that this endeavour is misplaced. Not only have no magic bullets been identified yet, but I also believe *they never will be identified* – and that we should stop looking for them.

This is because the implementation of best practice is highly complex; it involves multiple influences operating in different directions, [33] and it is dependent on *people*. An approach that has a positive effect in one study might have a negative effect in another study, so the notion of an 'effect size' of an intervention to change clinician behaviour is not only meaningless but also actively misleading. If you have children, you'll know that a strategy that worked well for your first child might not have worked at all for your second child, for reasons you can't easily explain. It's something to do with human quirkiness (child two is a different individual with a different personality), and also to do with the fact that the context is subtly different in multiple ways, even in the 'same' family environment (child two has an older sibling, busier parents, hand-me-down toys and so on). So it is with organisations, their staff and evidence-based practice. Even the more refined research approach of looking for 'mediators' and 'moderators' of the effectiveness of particular interventions [28] is still, in my view, based on the flawed assumption that there is a consistent 'mediator/moderator effect' from a particular contextual variable.

Let's think a bit more about the human factor. In a systematic review of the diffusion of organisational-level innovations in health services,

I drew this conclusion about the human elements in the adoption of innovations:

> People are not passive recipients of innovations. Rather (and to a greater or lesser extent in different individuals), they seek innovations out, experiment with them, evaluate them, find (or fail to find) meaning in them, develop feelings (positive or negative) about them, challenge them, worry about them, complain about them, 'work round' them, talk to others about them, develop know-how about them, modify them to fit particular tasks, and attempt to improve or redesign them.[8]

The key factors my team found to be associated with a person's readiness to adopt health care innovations were these:[8]

1 *General psychological antecedents*. A number of personality traits are associated with propensity to try out and use innovations (e.g. tolerance of ambiguity, intellectual ability, motivation, values and learning style). In short, some people are more set in their ways than others – and these individuals will need more input and take more time to change. For an amusing overview of strategies used by less innovative individuals to resist change, see Shaughnessy and Slawson's tongue-in-cheek review.[34]

2 *Context-specific psychological antecedents*. A person who is motivated and capable (in terms of values, goals, specific skills and so on) to use a particular innovation is more likely to adopt it. Also, if the innovation meets an *identified need* in the intended adopter, they are more likely to adopt it.

3 *Meaning*. The meaning that the innovation holds for the person has a powerful influence on his or her decision to adopt it. The meaning attached to an innovation is generally not fixed but can be negotiated and reframed – for example, through discussions with other professionals or others within the organization. For example, in the example described in Section 13.1, one of the problems was probably that dexamethasone therapy was unconsciously seen by doctors as 'an old-fashioned palliative care drug, mainly to be used in the elderly'. In changing their practice, they had to place this therapy in a new mental schema – as 'an up-to-date preventive therapy, appropriate for pregnant women'.

4 *Nature of the adoption decision*. The decision by an individual in an organization to adopt a particular innovation is rarely independent of other decisions. It may be contingent (dependent on a decision made by someone else in the organization); collective (the individual has a 'vote' but ultimately must follow to the decision of a group); or authoritative (the individual is told whether to adopt or not). A good example of promoting evidence-based practice through an authoritative adoption decision is the

development of hospital or practice formularies. Drugs of marginal value or poor cost-effectiveness ratio can be removed from the list of drugs that the hospital is prepared to pay for. But (as you may have discovered if you work with an imposed formulary), such policies also inhibit evidence-based practice because the innovator who is ahead of the game must wait (sometimes years) for a committee decision before implementing a new standard of practice.

5 *Concerns and information needs.* People are concerned about different things at different stages in the adoption of an innovation. Initially, they need *general information* (what is the new 'evidence-based' practice, what does it cost and how might it affect me?); in the early adoption stages they need *hands-on information* (how do I make it work in practice?), and as they become more confident in the new practice, they need *development and adaptation information* (can I adapt this practice a bit to suit my circumstances, and if so, how should I do that?).

Having explored the nature of human idiosyncrasy, another important factor to consider is the influence one person can have on another.[8] As Everett Rogers first demonstrated in relation to the adoption of agricultural innovations by Iowa farmers (who are perhaps even more set in their ways than doctors), interpersonal contact is the most powerful method of influence.[35] The main type of interpersonal influence relevant to the adoption of evidence-based practice is the *opinion leader*. We copy two sorts of people: people we look up to ('expert opinion leaders') and people we think are just like us ('peer opinion leaders').[8,36]

An opinion leader who is opposed to a new practice – or even one who is lukewarm and fails to back it – has a lot of potential wrecking power. But as Mary Thomson O'Brien and her team discovered in their systematic review of opinion leader intervention trials, just because a doctor is more likely to change his or her prescribing behaviour if a respected opinion leader has already changed, it doesn't necessarily follow that targeting opinion leaders (doctors nominated by other doctors as individuals they would consult or copy) with educational interventions will lead to a widespread change in prescribing practice.[37] This is probably because opinion leaders have minds of their own, and also because of the many other influences on practice apart from that one individual. Oxman's systematic review gives several examples of so-called social influence policies that, in reality, failed to influence.[12]

Another important model of interpersonal influence, which the pharmaceutical industry has shown to be highly effective, is one-to-one contact between doctors and drug company representatives (discussed in Chapter 6 and known in the United Kingdom as 'reps' and as detailers in the United States), whose influence on clinical behaviour may be so dramatic that they have been dubbed the 'stealth bombers' of medicine.[38] In the United States, this tactic has been harnessed by the government in what is known as *academic detailing*: the educator books in to see the physician in the same way as industry representatives, but in this case the 'rep' provides objective, complete and comparative information about a range of different drugs and encourages the clinician to adopt a critical approach to the evidence. Such a strategy can achieve dramatic short-term changes in practice, [39] but not all trials have shown the same level of impact. As ever, the intervention should not be seen as a panacea.

A final approach to note in relation to supporting implementation of evidence-based practice is the use of computerised decision support systems that incorporate the research evidence and can be accessed by the busy practitioner at the touch of a button. Dozens of these systems are currently being developed, piloted and tested in randomised controlled trials. Relatively few are in routine use. Since the last edition of this book, a major systematic review has been updated to cover 100 empirical studies.[40] Overall, around two-thirds of these studies demonstrated improved clinical performance in the decision support arm, with the best results being in drug dosing and active clinical care (e.g. management of asthma) and the worst results in diagnosis. Systems that included a spontaneous prompt (as opposed to requiring the clinician to activate the system) were the most effective.

However, note what I said earlier about the complexity of the implementation of EBM. I am sceptical of studies that attempt to say 'computer-based decision support is/is not effective' or 'computer-based decision support has an effect of X magnitude'. They work for some people in some circumstances, and our research energies should now be directed at refining what we can say about *what sort of* computerised decision support, *for whom* and *in what circumstances*.[41] As Taylor and Wyatt suggest, 'Poor design and a failure to consider the practicalities of clinical settings have perhaps hindered the take-up of decision-support systems, but such systems could never be designed to fit seamlessly into existing ways of working'.[42] Plenty more work to be done in that field, then.

13.3 What does an 'evidence-based organisation' look like?

'What does an organisation that promotes the adoption of (evidence based) innovations look like?' was one of the questions that my own team addressed in our systematic review of the literature on diffusion of organisational level innovations.[8] We found that, in general, an organization will assimilate a new product or practice more readily if it is large, mature (has been established a long time), functionally differentiated (i.e. divided into semi-autonomous departments and units), specialised (a well-developed division of labour, such as specialist services); if it has slack resources (money and staff) to channel into new projects and if it has decentralised decision-making structures (teams can work autonomously). But although dozens of studies (and five meta-analyses) have been undertaken on the size and structure of organisations, all these determinants account for less than 15% of the variation in organisations' ability to support innovation (and in many studies, they explain none of the variation at all). In other words, it's not usually the structure of the organisation that makes the critical difference in supporting EBM.

More important in our review were less easily measurable dimensions of the organisation – particularly something the organisational theorists call *absorptive capacity.* Absorptive capacity is defined as the organisation's ability to identify, capture, interpret, share, reframe and re-codify new knowledge, to link it with its own existing knowledge base, and to put it to appropriate use.[43] Prerequisites for absorptive capacity include the organization's existing knowledge and skills base (especially its store of tacit, 'knowing the ropes' type knowledge) and pre-existing related technologies; a 'learning organization' culture (in which people are encouraged to learn amongst themselves and share knowledge) and proactive leadership directed towards enabling this knowledge sharing.[44]

A major overview by Sue Dopson and her colleagues of high-quality qualit-ative studies on how research evidence is identified, circulated, evaluated and used in health care organizations[45] found that before it can be fully imple-mented in an organisation, EBM knowledge must be enacted and made social, entering into the stock of knowledge that is developed and socially shared amongst others in the organisation. In other words, knowledge depends for its circulation on interpersonal networks (who knows whom), and will only spread efficiently through the organisation if these social features are taken into account and barriers overcome.

Another difficult-to-measure dimension of the evidence-based organisa-tion (i.e. one that is capable of capturing best practice and implementing it widely in the organisation) is what is known as a *receptive context for change.* This composite construct, developed in relation to the implementation of best practice in health care by Pettigrew and McKee, [46] incorporates a num-ber of organizational features that have been independently associated with its ability to embrace new ideas and face the prospect of change. In addi-tion to absorptive capacity for new knowledge (see above), the components of receptive context include strong leadership, clear strategic vision, good managerial relations, visionary staff in key positions, a climate conducive to experimentation and risk taking, and effective data capture systems. Leadership may be especially critical in encouraging organizational members to break out of the convergent thinking and routines that are the norm in large, well-established organizations.[46]

Another paper that's worth looking up is Dave Gustafson's quasi-systematic review of the determinants of successful change projects in health care organisations.[47] The 18 items in Gustafson's final model include

1 tension for change (staff feel that current practice is suboptimal and want things to be different);

2 balance of power (staff supporting the change outnumber, and are more strategically placed in the organisation, than staff opposing it);

3 perceived advantages (everyone understands the change and believes its advantages outweigh the disadvantages);

4 flexibility (the new practice can be adapted to fit local needs and ways of working); and

5 time and resources (the change is adequately funded and people have protected time to work on it).

If this sounds like a recipe your organisation can't follow in relation to EBM, read the next section (and if that doesn't help, consider changing jobs!).

13.4 What evidence-based interventions are there for achieving organisational change to support evidence-based practice?

While there is a wealth of evidence on the sort of organisation that supports evidence-based practice, there is much less evidence on the effectiveness of specific interventions to *change* an organisation to make it more 'evidence based' – and it's beyond the scope of this book to address this topic comprehensively. Much of the literature on organisational change is in the form of practical checklists or the 'ten tips for success' type format. Checklists and tips can be enormously useful, but such lists can leave you hungry for some coherent conceptual models on which to hang your own real-life experiences.

The management literature offers not one but several dozen different conceptual frameworks for looking at change – leaving the non-expert confused about where to start. It was my attempt to make sense of this multiplicity of theories that led me to write a series of six articles published a few years ago in the *British Journal of General Practice* and entitled 'Theories of change'. In these articles, I explored six different models of professional and organisational change in relation to effective clinical practice:

1 *Adult learning theory*, the notion that adults learn via a cycle of thinking and doing. This explains why instructional education is so consistently

ineffective, and why hands-on practical experience with the opportunity to reflect and discuss with colleagues is the fundamental basis for both learning and change[48];

2 *Psychoanalytic theory*, Freud's famous concept of the unconscious, which influences (and sometimes overrides) our conscious, rational self. People's resistance to change can sometimes have powerful and deep-rooted emotional explanations[49];

3 *Group relations theory*, based on studies by specialists at London's Tavistock clinic on how teams operate (or fail to operate) in the work environment. Relationships both within the team and between the team and its wider environment can act as barriers to (or catalysts of) change[50];

4 *Anthropological theory*, the notion that organisations have cultures – that is, ways of doing things and of thinking about problems – that are, in general, highly resistant to change. A relatively minor proposed change towards evidence-based practice (such as requiring consultants to look up evidence routinely on the Cochrane database) may in reality be highly threatening to the culture of the organisation (in which, e.g. the 'consultant opinion' has traditionally carried an almost priestly status)[51];

5 *Classical management theory*, the notion that 'mainstreaming' a change within an organisation requires a systematic plan to make it happen. The vision for change must be shared amongst a critical mass of staff, and must be accompanied by planned changes to the visible structures of the organisation, to the roles and responsibilities of key individuals, and to information and communication systems[52];

6 *Complexity theory*, the notion that large organisations (such as the UK National Health Service) depend critically on the dynamic, evolving and local relationships and communication systems between individuals. Supporting key interpersonal relationships and improving the quality and timeliness of information available locally are often more crucial factors in achieving sustained change than 'top down' directives or overarching national or regional programmes.[53]

There are, as I have said, many additional models of change that might come in useful when identifying and overcoming barriers to achieving evidence-based practice. The list above is not intended to be exhaustive – and given the complex nature of health care organisations, none of them will provide a simple formula for successful change.

I would now add a seventh theoretical model to the above list – that of change as a *social movement*, that is, as a powerful groundswell of activity that is bound up with individuals' identity as part of the movement for change. If you've ever been on a protest march, or joined a residents' initiative to improve some local service or other, you'll know what it feels like to be part of a social movement. I was once on a high-level committee that tried to close the little-used casualty department of a small hospital on the grounds that there was no evidence that it was either effective or cost-effective – but I bargained without the input of the 'Hands Off Our Hospital' campaign. Indeed, many successful changes in clinical practice towards evidence-based care (e.g. the abolition of routine episiotomy in obstetric care) were achieved primarily through patient pressure groups operating in 'social movement' mode.

The interesting thing about social movements for change is that while they can achieve profound and widespread change, they can't be planned, controlled or their behaviour predicted in the same way as a conventional management model. For an outstanding summary of the literature on social movements for change in health care, see Paul Bate and colleagues' booklet.[54] You might also like to look at Cathy Pope's sociological analysis of the rise of EBM as a social movement![55]

Whatever theoretical approach you take to change, converting your theories into practice will be a tough challenge. A publication by the UK National Association of Health Authorities and Trusts (NAHAT), entitled 'Acting on the evidence', emphasises that the task of supporting and empowering managers and clinical professionals to use evidence as part of their everyday decision making is massive and complex.[56] An action checklist for health care organisations working towards an evidence-based culture for clinical and policy-making decisions, listed at the end of Appendix 1, is adapted from the NAHAT report.

First and foremost, key players within the organisation, particularly chief executives, board members and senior clinicians, must create an evidence-based culture where decision making is *expected* to be based on the best available evidence. High-quality, up-to-date information sources (such as the Cochrane electronic library and the Medline database) should be available in every office, and staff given protected time to access them. Ideally, users should only have to deal with a single access point for all available sources. Information on the clinical and cost-effectiveness of particular technologies should be produced, disseminated and used together. Individuals who collate and disseminate this information within the organisation need to be aware of who will use it and how it will be applied – and tailor their presentation accordingly. They should also set standards for, and evaluate, the quality of the evidence they are circulating. Individuals on the organisation's internal mailing list for effectiveness information need training and support if they are to make the best use of this information.

This sound advice from NAHAT is based (implicitly if not explicitly) on the notion of the *learning organisation*. As Davies and Nutley have pointed out,

'Learning is something achieved by individuals, but "learning organisations" can configure themselves to maximise, mobilise, and retain this learning potential'.[57] Drawing on the work of Senge,[58] they offer five key features of a learning organisation:

1 People are encouraged to move beyond traditional professional or departmental boundaries (an approach Senge called 'open systems thinking').

2 Individuals' personal learning needs are systematically identified and addressed.

3 Learning occurs to some extent in teams, since it is largely through teams that organisations achieve their objectives.

4 Efforts are made to change the way people conceptualise issues – hence allowing new, creative approaches to old problems.

5 Senior clinicians and managers provide leadership to drive through a shared vision with coherent values and clear strategic direction, so that staff willingly pull together towards a common goal.

Turning a traditional organisation into a learning organisation is a tough task, which often involves a major shift in organisational culture (the unwritten rules, assumptions and expectations that make up 'how things are done around here'). While it's not possible for any single individual to turn an organisation around, if you're sufficiently senior to write the job description of a new member of staff, or to decide how a training budget is spent or to choose who is involved in a key decision, you can start to move your organisation in the right direction (see Table 13.2).

A core principle in developing a learning organisation is to *invest in people*. In addition to strong leadership from the top, some particular roles that you might think of supporting in relation to EBM include[8]

1 *Knowledge managers.* These are senior people hired not just to get the information systems right but to encourage the rest of us to use them. They make the decisions about what software licences to purchase for the organisation and which members of staff are allowed to access which knowledge sources. When I wrote the first edition of this book in 1995, a minority of hospitals had a rule that staff nurses couldn't go into the medical library or dial up an Internet connection. The role of the knowledge manager is to blow this sort of nonsense away and ensure that (in the case of EBM) everyone who needs to practice it has links to the relevant knowledge base, protected time to access it and appropriate training.

2 *Knowledge workers.* These individuals have it on their job description to help the rest of us find and apply knowledge. The person on the computer helpdesk is a kind of knowledge worker, as is a librarian or a research assistant. To use some contemporary jargon, the tools of EBM should be

offered as an 'augmented product' with designated members of staff hired
to provide flexible support to individuals as and when they ask for it.
3 *Champions.* Adoption of a new practice by individuals in an organization
or professional group is more likely if key individuals within that group
are willing to back the innovation. 'Backing' an evidence-based innovation
might include, for example, talking enthusiastically about it, showing
people how to use it, getting it on the agenda of key committees, giving staff
protected time to learn about it and try it out and rewarding people who
take it up. While there's remarkably little research evidence about what
champions actually do (or what's the most effective way of championing an
evidence-based change), the principle is pretty simple: designate particular
individuals at every level in your organisation to back it.
4 *Boundary spanners.* An organization is more likely to adopt a new approach
to practice if individuals can be identified who have significant social ties
both within and outside the organization, and who are able and willing
to link the organization to the outside world in relation to this particular
practice. Such individuals play a pivotal role in capturing the ideas that
will become organizational innovations. If you've got a member of staff
who is well connected in relation to an aspect of evidence-based practice,
make a point of drawing on their connections and expertise. Send staff
out of the organisation – on conferences, visits to comparable organisations or to quality improvement collaboratives – and when they return,
capture what they've learnt by making time to listen to their stories and
ideas.

A specific tool to consider when working towards the 'evidence-based organisation' is the idea of *integrated care pathways*, defined as pre-defined plans
of patient care relating to a specific diagnosis (e.g. suspected fractured hip)
or intervention (e.g. hernia repair), with the aim of making the management
more structured, consistent and efficient.[59] A good care pathway integrates
evidence-based recommendations with the realities of local services, usually
via a multi-professional initiative that engages both clinicians and managers.
The care pathway states not only what intervention is recommended at different stages in the course of the condition, but also whose responsibility it is
to undertake the task and to follow up if it gets missed. While there are many
care pathways in circulation (see e.g. the UK National Electronic Library for
Health on www.nelh.org.uk for an archive of downloadable ones), it is often
the process of developing the pathway as much as the finished product that
engages staff across the organisation to focus on evidence-based care in the
target condition. If your organisation is resistant to the whole concept of
EBM, you might find that the process of developing one care pathway for a
relatively uncontroversial condition builds a surprising amount of goodwill

Table 13.2 Key differences between a traditional organisation and a learning organisation

Feature	Traditional organisation	Learning organisation
Organisational boundaries	Clearly demarcated	Permeable
Structure of the organisation	Pre-designed and fixed	Evolving
Approach to human resources	Minimum skill set to do the job	Maximise skills to enhance creativity and learning
Approach to complex activities	Divide into segmented tasks	Ensure integrated processes
Divisions and departments	Functional, hierarchical groupings	Open, multifunctional networks

Adapted from Senge – see reference 58.

and buy-in to the principle of evidence-based practice, which can be drawn upon in rolling out the idea more widely.

Finally, note that the UK Department of Health's Service Delivery and Organisation Programme (see www.nhssdo.org) is funding an exciting collection of empirical studies on the development, delivery and organisation of health services, many of them highly relevant to the implementation of best practice at organisational level.

13.5 Why is it so hard to get evidence into policy making?

The main reason why policies don't flow simply and logically from research evidence is that there are so many other factors involved.

Take the question of publicly funded treatments for infertility, for example. You can produce a stack of evidence as high as a house to demonstrate that intervention X leads to a take-home baby rate of $Y\%$ in women with characteristics (such as age or comorbidity) Z, but that won't take the heat out of the decision to sanction infertility treatment from a limited health care budget. This was the question addressed by a Primary Care Trust policy-making forum I attended recently, which had to balance this decision against competing options (outreach support for first episode of psychosis and a community-based diabetes specialist nurse for epilepsy). It wasn't that the members of the forum ignored the evidence – there was so much evidence in the background papers that the courier couldn't get it to fit through my letterbox – it was that values, rather than evidence, were what the final decision hung on. And as Nick Black and Cindy Mulrow have pointed out in editorials,[60,61] policy making is as much about the struggle to resolve conflicts of values in particular local or national contexts as it is about getting evidence into practice.

In other words, the policy-making process cannot be considered as a 'macro' version of the sequence depicted in Section 1.1 ('convert our information needs into answerable questions...' etc.). Like other processes that fall under the heading 'politics' (with a small 'p'), policy making is fundamentally about *persuading* one's fellow decision makers of the superiority of one course of action over another. This model of the policy-making process is strongly supported by research studies, which suggest that at its heart lies unpredictability, ambiguity and the possibility of alternative interpretations of the 'evidence'.[62–65]

The quest to make policy making 'fully evidence based' may actually not be a desirable goal, since this benchmark arguably devalues democratic debate about the ethical and moral issues faced in policy choices. The 2005 UK Labour Party manifesto claimed that 'what matters is what works'. But what matters, surely, is not just what 'works', but what is appropriate in the circumstances and what is agreed by society to be the overall desirable goal. Deborah Stone, in her book *Policy paradox*, argues that much of the policy process involves debates about values masquerading as debates about facts and data. In her words: 'The essence of policymaking in political communities [is] the struggle over ideas. Ideas are at the centre of all political conflict ...Each idea is an argument, or more accurately, a collection of arguments in favour of different ways of seeing the world.'[66]

One of the most useful theoretical papers on the use of evidence in health care policy making is by Mark Dobrow and colleagues.[67] They distinguish the philosophical–normative orientation (that there is an objective reality to be discovered and that a piece of 'evidence' can be deemed 'valid' and 'reliable' independent of the context in which it is to be used) from the practical–operational orientation, in which evidence is defined in relation to a specific decision-making context, is never static and is characterized by emergence, ambiguity and incompleteness. From a practical–operational standpoint, research evidence is based on designs (such as randomized trials) that explicitly strip the study of contextual 'contaminants' and which therefore ignore the multiple, complex and interacting determinants of health. It follows that a complex intervention that 'works' in one setting at one time will not necessarily 'work' in a different setting at a different time, and one that proves 'cost-effective' in one setting will not necessarily provide value for money in a different setting. Many of the arguments raised about EBM in recent years have addressed precisely this controversy about the nature of knowledge.

Questioning the nature of evidence – and indeed, questioning evidential knowledge itself – is a somewhat scary place to end a basic introductory textbook on EBM, since the previous 12 chapters in this book assume what Dobrow would call a philosophical–normative orientation. My own advice is this: if you are a humble student or clinician trying to pass your exams or do a better job at the bedside of individual patients, and if you feel thrown by the uncertainties I've raised in this final section, you can probably safely ignore them until you're actively involved in policy making yourself. But if your career is at the stage when you're already sitting on decision-making bodies and trying to work out the answer to the question posed in the title to this section, I'd suggest you explore some of the papers and books referenced below. Do watch for the next generation of EBM research, which increasingly addresses the fuzzier and more contestible aspects of EBM.

References

1 Van Someren V. Changing clinical practice in the light of the evidence: two contrasting stories from perinatology. In: *Getting research findings into practice*. London: BMJ Publications, 1998.

2 NIH Consensus Development Panel on the Effect of Corticosteroids for Fetal Maturation on Perinatal Outcomes. Effect of corticosteroids for fetal maturation on perinatal outcomes. *JAMA* 1995;273:413–18.

3 Halliday HL. Overview of clinical trials comparing natural and synthetic surfactants. *Biol Neonate* 1995;67:32–47.

4 Crowley P. Prophylactic corticosteroids for preterm birth. *Cochrane Database of Systematic Reviews* 2000;(2):CD000065.

5 Booth-Clibborn N, Packer C, Stevens A. Health technology diffusion rates. Statins, coronary stents, and MRI in England. *Int J Technol Assess Health Care* 2000;16:781–6.

6 Granados A, Jonsson E, Banta HD, Bero L, Bonair A, Cochet C *et al.* EUR-ASSESS project subgroup report on dissemination and impact. *Int J Technol Assess Health Care* 1997;13:220–86.

7 Drummond M, Weatherly H. Implementing the findings of health technology assessments. If the CAT got out of the bag, can the TAIL wag the dog? *Int J Technol Assess Health Care* 2000;16:1–12.

8 Greenhalgh T, Robert G, Macfarlane F, Bate P, Kyriakidou O. Diffusion of innovations in service organisations: systematic literature review and recommendations for future research. *Milbank Q* 2004;82:581–629.

9 Mowatt G, Grimshaw JM, Davis DA, Mazmanian PE. Getting evidence into practice: the work of the Cochrane Effective Practice and Organization of care Group (EPOC). *J Contin Educ Health Prof* 2001;**21**:55–60.

10 Stanton F, Grant J. *The effectiveness of continuing professional development.* London: Joint Centre for Medical Education, Open University, 1997.

11 Davis DA, Thomson MA, Oxman AD, Haynes RB. Changing physician performance. A systematic review of the effect of continuing medical education strategies. *JAMA* 1995;**274**:700–5.

12 Oxman AD, Thomson MA, Davis DA, Haynes RB. No magic bullets: a systematic review of 102 trials of interventions to improve professional practice. *CMAJ* 1995;**153**:1423–31.

13 Caulford PG, Lamb SB, Kaigas TB, Hanna E, Norman GR, Davis DA. Physician incompetence: specific problems and predictors. *Acad Med* 1994;**69**: S16–S18.

14 Marteau T, Snowden A, Armstrong D. Implementing research findings in practice: beyond the information deficit model. In: Haines A, Donald A, eds. *Getting research findings into practice.* London: BMJ Publications, 1998:36–42.

15 Norman GR, Shannon SI. Effectiveness of instruction in critical appraisal (evidence-based medicine) skills: a critical appraisal. *CMAJ* 1998;**158**: 177–81.

16 Taylor R, Reeves B, Ewings P, Binns S, Keast J, Mears R. A systematic review of the effectiveness of critical appraisal skills training for clinicians. *Med Educ* 2000;**34**:120–5.

17 Parkes J, Hyde C, Deeks J, Milne R. Teaching critical appraisal skills in health care settings. *Cochrane Database Syst Rev* 2001;CD001270.

18 Welch HG, Lurie JD. Teaching evidence-based medicine: caveats and challenges. *Acad Med* 2000;**75**:235–40.

19 Green ML. Evidence-based medicine training in graduate medical education: past, present and future. *J Eval Clin Pract* 2000;**6**:121–38.

20 Fritsche L, Greenhalgh T, Falck-Ytter Y, Neumayer HH, Kunz R. Do short courses in evidence based medicine improve knowledge and skills? Validation of Berlin questionnaire and before and after study of courses in evidence based medicine. *BMJ* 2002;**325**:1338–41.

21 Norman GR, Shannon SI. Effectiveness of instruction in critical appraisal (evidence-based medicine) skills: a critical appraisal. *CMAJ* 1998;**158**:177–81.

22 Dobbie AE, Schneider FD, Anderson AD, Littlefield J. What evidence supports teaching evidence-based medicine? *Acad Med* 2000;**75**:1184–5.

23 Green ML. Graduate medical education training in clinical epidemiology, critical appraisal and evidence-based medicine: a critical review of curricula. *Acad Med* 1999;**74**:686–94.

24 Green ML. Evidence based medicine training in internal medicine residency programs a national survey. *J Gen Intern Med* 2000;**6**:121–38.

25 Green ML. Evidence-based medicine training in graduate medical education: past, present and future. *J Eval Clin Pract* 2000;**6**:121–38.

26 Sackett D, Straus SE. Finding and applying evidence during clinical rounds: the 'evidence cart'. *JAMA* 1998;**280**:1336–8.

27 Eccles M, Grimshaw J, Walker A, Johnston M, Pitts N. Changing the behavior of healthcare professionals: the use of theory in promoting the uptake of research findings. *J Clin Epidemiol* 2005;**58**:107–12.

28 Grimshaw JM, Thomas RE, MacLennan G, Fraser C, Ramsay CR, Vale L, Whitty P, Eccles MP, Matowe L, Shirran L, Wensing M, Dikstra R, Donaldson C and Hutchinson A. Effectiveness and efficiency of guideline dissemination and implementation strategies. *Health Technol Assess Rep* 2004;**8**(6):1–72.

29 Grol R. Personal paper. Beliefs and evidence in changing clinical practice. *BMJ* 1997;**315**:418–21.

30 Freemantle N, Harvey EL, Wolf F, Grimshaw JM, Grilli R, Bero LA. Printed educational materials: effects on professional practice and health care outcomes. *Cochrane Database Syst Rev* 2000;CD000172.

31 Thomson O'Brien MA, Oxman AD, Davis DA, Haynes RB, Freemantle N, Harvey EL. Audit and feedback: effects on professional practice and health care outcomes. *Cochrane Database Syst Rev* 2000;CD000259.

32 Giuffrida A, Gosden T, Forland F, Kristiansen IS, Sergison M, Leese B *et al.* Target payments in primary care: effects on professional practice and health care outcomes. *Cochrane Database Syst Rev* 2000;CD000531.

33 Plsek PE, Greenhalgh T. Complexity science: the challenge of complexity in health care. *BMJ* 2001;**323**:625–8.

34 Shaughnessy AF, Slawson DC. Easy ways to resist change in medicine. *BMJ* 2004;**329**:1473–4.

35 Rogers EM. *Diffusion of innovations.* New York: Free Press, 1995.

36 Locock L, Dopson S, Chambers D, Gabbay J. Understanding the role of opinion leaders in improving clinical effectiveness. *Soc Sci Med* 2001;**53**:745–57.

37 Thomson O'Brien MA, Oxman AD, Haynes RB, Davis DA, Freemantle N, Harvey EL. Local opinion leaders: effects on professional practice and health care outcomes. *Cochrane Database Syst Rev* 2000;CD000125.

38 Shaughnessy AF, Slawson DC. Pharmaceutical representatives. *BMJ* 2005;**312**:1494–5.

39 Thomson O'Brien MA, Oxman AD, Davis DA, Haynes RB, Freemantle N, Harvey EL. Educational outreach visits: effects on professional practice and health care outcomes. *Cochrane Database Syst Rev* 2000;CD000409.

40 Garg AX, Adhikari NK, McDonald H, Rosas-Arellano MP, Devereaux PJ, Beyene J *et al.* Effects of computerized clinical decision support systems on practitioner performance and patient outcomes: a systematic review. *JAMA* 2005;**293**:1223–38.

41 Pawson R, Greenhalgh T, Harvey G, Walshe K. Realist review – a new method of systematic review designed for complex policy interventions. *J Health Serv Res Policy* 2005;**10**(Suppl 1):21–34.

42 Taylor P, Wyatt JC. Decision support. In: Haines A, Donald A, eds. *Getting research findings into practice.* London: BMJ Publications, 1998.

43 Zahra AS, George G. Absorptive capacity: a review, reconceptualization and extension. *Acad Manage Rev* 2002;**27**:185–203.

44 Ferlie E, Gabbay J, Fitzgerald L, Locock L, Dopson S. Evidence-based medicine and organisational change: an overview of some recent qualitative research. In: Ashburner L, ed. *Organisational behaviour and organisational studies in health care: reflections on the future.* Basingstoke: Palgrave, 2001.

45 Dopson S, Fitzgerald L, Ferlie E, Gabbay J, Locock L. No magic targets. Changing clinical practice to become more evidence based. *Health Care Manage Rev* 2002;**37**:35–47.

46 Pettigrew AM, McKee L. *Shaping strategic change. Making change in large organisations.* London: Sage, 1992.

47 Gustafson DH, Sainfort F, Eichler M, Adams L, Bisognano M, Steudel H. Developing and testing a model to predict outcomes of organizational change. *Health Serv Res* 2003;**38**:751–76.

48 Greenhalgh T. Change and the individual 1: Adult learning theory. *Br J Gen Pract* 2000;**50**:76–7.

49 Greenhalgh T. Change and the individual 2: psychoanalytic theory. *Br J Gen Pract* 2000;**50**:164–5.

50 Greenhalgh T. Change and the team: group relations theory. *Br J Gen Pract* 2000;**50**:262–3.

51 Greenhalgh T. Change and the organisation 1: culture and context. *Br J Gen Pract* 2000;**50**:340–1.

52 Greenhalgh T. Change and the organisation 2: strategy. *Br J Gen Pract* 2000;**50**:424–5.

53 Greenhalgh T. Change and complexity: the rich picture. *Br J Gen Pract* 2000;**50**:514–15.

54 Bate SP, Bevan H, Robert G. *Towards a million change agents: a review of the social movements literature.* London: NHS SDO Programme, 2005.

55 Pope C. Resisting evidence: a study of evidence based medicine as a contemporary social movement. *Health: An Interdisciplinary J Soc Stud Health Illn Med* 2003;**7**:267–82.

56 Appleby J, Walshe K, Ham C. Acting on the evidence: a review of clinical effectiveness: sources of information, dissemination and implementation. Birmingham: National Association of Health Authorities and Trusts, 1995.

57 Davies HTO, Nutley SM. Developing learning organisations in the new NHS. *BMJ* 2000;**320**:998–1001.

58 Senge PM. *The fifth discipline – the art and practice of the learning organisation.* New York: Random House Business Books, 1993.

59 Renholm M, Leino-Kilpi H, Suominen T. Critical pathways. A systematic review. *J Nurs Adm* 2002;**32**:196–202.

60 Black N. Evidence based policy: proceed with care. *BMJ* 2001;**323**:275–9.

61 Mulrow CD, Lohr KN. Proof and policy from medical research evidence. *J Health Polit Policy Law* 2001;**26**:249–66.

62 Elliott H, Popay J. How are policy makers using evidence? Models of research utilisation and local NHS policy making. *J Epidemiol Community Health* 2000;**54**:461–8.

63 Innvaer S, Vist G, Trommald M, Oxman A. Health policy-makers' perceptions of their use of evidence: a systematic review. *J Health Serv Res Policy* 2002;**7**:239–44.

64 Lavis JN, Ross SE, Hurley JE, Hohenadel JM, Stoddart GL, Woodward CA *et al.* Examining the role of health services research in public policymaking. *Milbank Q* 2002;**80**:125–54.

65 Scheel IB, Hagen KB, Oxman AD. The unbearable lightness of healthcare policy making: a description of a process aimed at giving it some weight. *J Epidemiol Community Health* 2003;**57**:483–7.

66 Stone D. *Policy paradox: the art of political decision making.* New York: W W Norton, 1997.

67 Dobrow MJ, Goel V, Upshur RE. Evidence-based health policy: context and utilisation. *Soc Sci Med* 2004;**58**:207–17.

Appendix 1 **Checklists for finding, appraising and implementing evidence**

Unless otherwise stated, these checklists can be applied to randomised controlled trials, other controlled clinical trials, cohort studies, case-control studies or any other research evidence.

Is my practice evidence based? – a context-sensitive checklist for individual clinical encounters (see Chapter 1)

1 Have I identified and prioritised the clinical, psychological, social and other problem(s), taking into account the patient's perspective?
2 Have I performed a sufficiently competent and complete examination to establish the likelihood of competing diagnoses?
3 Have I considered additional problems and risk factors which may need opportunistic attention?
4 Have I, where necessary, sought evidence (from systematic reviews, guidelines, clinical trials and other sources) pertaining to the problems?
5 Have I assessed and taken into account the completeness, quality and strength of the evidence?
6 Have I applied valid and relevant evidence to this particular set of problems in a way that is both scientifically justified and intuitively sensible?
7 Have I presented the pros and cons of different options to the patient in a way they can understand and incorporated the patient's utilities into the final recommendation?
8 Have I arranged review, recall, referral or other further care as necessary?

Checklist for searching Medline or the Cochrane library (see Chapter 2)

1 To look for an article that you know exists, search by textwords (in title, abstract or both), or use field suffixes for author, title, institution, journal and publication year.
2 For a maximally sensitive search on a subject, search under both MeSH headings (exploded) and textwords (title and abstract), then combine the two using the Boolean operator OR.

3 For a focused (specific) search on a clear-cut topic, perform two or more sensitive searches as in (2), and combine them using the Boolean operator AND.

4 To find articles which are likely to be of high methodological quality, insert an evidence-based filter or use databases of pre-appraised or pre-synthesised sources.

5 Refine your search as you go along. For example, to exclude irrelevant material, use the Boolean operator NOT.

6 Use subheadings only when this is the only practicable way of limiting your search, since manual indexers are fallible and misclassifications are common.

7 When limiting a large set, browse through the last 50 or so abstracts yourself rather than expecting the software to pick the best half-dozen.

Checklist to determine what a paper is about (see Chapter 3)

1 Why was the study done (what clinical question did it address)?

2 What type of study was done?
   a) Primary research (experiment, randomised controlled trial, other controlled clinical trial, cohort study, case-control study, cross-sectional survey, longitudinal survey, case report or case series)?
   b) Secondary research (simple overview, systematic review, meta-analysis, decision analysis, guideline development, economic analysis)?

3 Was the study design appropriate to the broad field of research addressed (therapy, diagnosis, screening, prognosis, causation)?

4 Did the study meet expected standards of ethics and governance?

Checklist for the methods section of a paper (see Chapter 4)

1 Was the study original?

2 Whom is the study about?
   a) How were participants recruited?
   b) Who was included in, and who was excluded from, the study?
   c) Were the participants studied in 'real life' circumstances?

3 Was the design of the study sensible?
   a) What intervention or other manoeuvre was being considered?
   b) What outcome(s) were measured, and how?

4 Was the study adequately controlled?
   a) If a 'randomised trial', was randomisation truly random?
   b) If a cohort, case-control or other non-randomised comparative study, were the controls appropriate?
   c) Were the groups comparable in all important aspects except for the variable being studied?

d) Was assessment of outcome (or, in a case-control study, allocation of caseness) 'blind'?

5 Was the study large enough, and continued for long enough, and was follow-up complete enough, to make the results credible?

Checklist for the statistical aspects of a paper (see Chapter 5)

1 Have the authors set the scene correctly?
   a) Have they determined whether their groups are comparable, and, if necessary, adjusted for baseline differences?
   b) What sort of data have they got, and have they used appropriate statistical tests?
   c) If the statistical tests in the paper are obscure, why have the authors chosen to use them?
   d) Have the data been analysed according to the original study protocol?
2 Paired data, tails and outliers
   a) Were paired tests performed on paired data?
   b) Was a two-tailed test performed whenever the effect of an intervention could conceivably be a negative one?
   c) Were outliers analysed with both common sense and appropriate statistical adjustments?
3 Correlation, regression and causation
   a) Has correlation been distinguished from regression, and has the correlation coefficient ('r-value') been calculated and interpreted correctly?
   b) Have assumptions been made about the nature and direction of causality?
4 Probability and confidence
   a) Have 'p-values' been calculated and interpreted appropriately?
   b) Have confidence intervals been calculated and do the authors' conclusions reflect them?
5 Have the authors expressed their results in terms of the likely harm or benefit which an individual patient can expect, such as
   a) relative risk reduction;
   b) absolute risk reduction;
   c) number needed to treat; or
   d) odds ratio?

Checklist for material provided by a pharmaceutical company representative (see Chapter 6)

1 Does this material cover a subject which interests me and is clinically important in my practice?

2 Has this material been published in independent peer-reviewed journals? Has any significant evidence been omitted from this presentation or withheld from publication?

3 Does the material include high-level evidence such as systematic reviews, meta-analyses or double-blind randomised controlled trials against the drug's closest competitor given at optimal dosage?

4 Have the trials or reviews addressed a clearly focused, important and answerable clinical question which reflects a problem of relevance to patients? Do they provide evidence on safety, tolerability, efficacy and price?

5 Has each trial or meta-analysis defined the condition to be treated, the patients to be included, the interventions to be compared and the outcomes to be examined?

6 Does the material provide direct evidence that the drug will help my patients live a longer, healthier, more productive and symptom-free life?

7 If a surrogate outcome measure has been used, what is the evidence that it is reliable, reproducible, sensitive, specific, a true predictor of disease and rapidly reflects the response to therapy?

8 Do trial results indicate whether (and how) the effectiveness of the treatments differed and whether there was a difference in the type or frequency of adverse reactions? Are the results expressed in terms of numbers needed to treat, and are they clinically as well as statistically significant?

9 If large amounts of material have been provided by the representative, which three papers provide the strongest evidence for the company's claims?

Checklist for a paper that claims to validate a diagnostic or screening test (see Chapter 7)

1 Is this test potentially relevant to my practice?

2 Has the test been compared with a true gold standard?

3 Did this validation study include an appropriate spectrum of participants?

4 Has workup bias been avoided?

5 Has observer bias been avoided?

6 Was the test shown to be reproducible both within and between observers?

7 What are the features of the test as derived from this validation study?

8 Were confidence intervals given for sensitivity, specificity and other features of the test?

9 Has a sensible 'normal range' been derived from these results?

10 Has this test been placed in the context of other potential tests in the diagnostic sequence for the condition?

Checklist for a systematic review or meta-analysis (see Chapter 8)

1 Did the review address an important clinical question?
2 Was a thorough search done of the appropriate database(s) and were other potentially important sources explored?
3 Was methodological quality assessed and the trials weighted accordingly?
4 How sensitive are the results to the way the review has been done?
5 Have the numerical results been interpreted with common sense and due regard to the broader aspects of the problem?

Checklist for a set of clinical guidelines (see Chapter 9)

1 Did the preparation and publication of these guidelines involve a significant conflict of interest?
2 Are the guidelines concerned with an appropriate topic, and do they state clearly the goal of ideal treatment in terms of health and/or cost outcome?
3 Was a specialist in the methodology of secondary research (e.g. meta-analyst) involved?
4 Have all the relevant data been scrutinised and are guidelines' conclusions in keeping with the data?
5 Do they address variations in clinical practice and other controversial areas (e.g. optimum care in response to genuine or perceived underfunding)?
6 Are the guidelines valid and reliable?
7 Are they clinically relevant, comprehensive and flexible?
8 Do they take into account what is acceptable to, affordable by and practically possible for patients?
9 Do they include recommendations for their own dissemination, implementation and periodic review?

Checklist for an economic analysis (see Chapter 10)

1 Is the analysis based on a study which answers a clearly defined clinical question about an economically important issue?
2 Whose viewpoint are costs and benefits being considered from?
3 Have the interventions being compared been shown to be clinically effective?
4 Are the interventions sensible and workable in the settings where they are likely to be applied?
5 Which method of economic analysis was used, and was this appropriate?
   a) If the interventions produced identical outcomes ⇒ cost-minimisation analysis.
   b) If the important outcome is unidimensional ⇒ cost-effectiveness analysis.

c) If the important outcome is multidimensional $\Rightarrow$ cost–utility analysis.

d) If the cost–benefit equation for this condition needs to be compared with cost–benefit equations for different conditions $\Rightarrow$ cost–benefit analysis.

e) If a cost–benefit analysis would otherwise be appropriate but the preference values given to different health states are disputed or likely to change $\Rightarrow$ cost–consequences analysis.

6 How were costs and benefits measured?

7 Were incremental, rather than absolute, benefits compared?

8 Was health status in the 'here and now' given precedence over health status in the distant future?

9 Was a sensitivity analysis performed?

10 Were 'bottom line' aggregate scores overused?

Checklist for a qualitative research paper (see Chapter 11)

1 Did the article describe an important clinical problem addressed via a clearly formulated question?

2 Was a qualitative approach appropriate?

3 How were (a) the setting and (b) the participants selected?

4 What was the researcher's perspective, and has this been taken into account?

5 What methods did the researcher use for collecting data – and are these described in enough detail?

6 What methods did the researcher use to analyse the data – and what quality control measures were implemented?

7 Are the results credible, and if so, are they clinically important?

8 What conclusions were drawn, and are they justified by the results?

9 Are the findings of the study transferable to other clinical settings?

Checklist for a paper describing questionnaire research (see Chapter 12)

1 What did the researchers want to find out, and was a questionnaire the most appropriate research design?

2 If an 'off the peg' questionnaire (i.e. a previously published and validated one) was available, did the researchers use it (and if not, why not)?

3 What claims have the researchers made about the validity of the questionnaire (its ability to measure what they want it to measure) and reliability (its ability to give consistent results across time and within/between researchers)? Are these claims justified?

4 Was the questionnaire appropriately structured and presented, and were the items worded appropriately for the sensitivity of the subject area and the health literacy of the respondents?
5 Were adequate instructions and explanations included?
6 Was the questionnaire adequately piloted, and was the definitive version amended in the light of pilot results?
7 Was the sample of potential participants appropriately selected, large enough and representative enough?
8 How was the questionnaire distributed (e.g. by post, email, telephone) and administered (self-completion, researcher-assisted completion), and were these approaches appropriate?
9 Were the needs of particular subgroups taken into account in the design and administration of the questionnaire? For example, what was done to capture the perspective of illiterate respondents or those speaking a different language form the researcher?
10 What was the response rate, and why? If the response rate was low (less than 70%), have the researchers shown that no systematic differences existed between responders and non-responders?
11 What sort of analysis was carried out on the questionnaire data, and was this appropriate? Is there any evidence of 'data dredging' – that is, analyses that were not hypothesis driven?
12 What were the results? Were they definitive (statistically significant), and were important negative and non-significant results also reported?
13 Have qualitative data (e.g. free text responses) been adequately interpreted (e.g. using an explicit theoretical framework). Have quotes been used judiciously to illustrate more general findings rather than to add drama?
14 What do the results mean and have the researchers drawn an appropriate link between the data and their conclusions?

Checklist for health care organisations working towards an evidence-based culture for clinical and purchasing decisions (see Chapter 13)

1 *Leadership.* How often has effectiveness information or evidence-based medicine been discussed at board meetings in the last 12 months? Has the board taken time out to learn about developments in clinical and cost-effectiveness?
2 *Investment.* What resources is the organisation investing in finding and using clinical effectiveness information? Is there a planned approach to promoting evidence-based medicine which is properly resourced and staffed?

3 *Policies and guidelines.* Who is responsible for receiving, acting on and monitoring the implementation of evidence-based guidance and policy recommendations such as NICE guidance or Effective Health Care Bulletins? What action has been taken on each of these publications issued to date? Do arrangements ensure that both managers and clinicians play their part in guideline development and implementation?

4 *Training.* Has any training been provided to staff within the organisation (both clinical and non-clinical) on appraising and using evidence of effectiveness to influence clinical practice?

5 *Contracts.* How often does clinical and cost-effectiveness information form an important part of contract negotiation and agreement? How many contracts contain terms which set out how effectiveness information is to be used?

6 *Incentives.* What incentives – both individual and organisational – exist to encourage the practice of evidence-based medicine? What disincentives exist to discourage inappropriate practice and unjustified variations in clinical decision making?

7 *Information systems.* Is the potential of existing information systems to monitor clinical effectiveness being used to the full? Is there a business case for new information systems to address the task, and is this issue being considered when IT purchasing decisions are made?

8 *Clinical audit.* Is there an effective clinical audit programme throughout the organisation, capable of addressing issues of clinical effectiveness and bringing about appropriate changes in practice?

Appendix 2 **Assessing the effects of an intervention**

Let's assume we are looking at the results of an intervention trial aimed at reducing the incidence of an undesirable event (such as death). The results could be expressed in a 2×2 table as follows:

	Outcome event		Total
	Yes	No	
Control group	a	b	$a + b$
Experimental group	c	d	$c + d$

Control event rate = risk of outcome event in control group = CER = a/(a+b)

Experimental event rate = risk of outcome event in experimental group = EER = $c/(c + d)$

Absolute risk reduction (ARR) = EER − CER

Relative risk reduction (RRR) = (EER − CER)/CER

Number needed to treat (NNT) = 1/ARR = 1/(CER − EER)

Odds ratio for a particular outcome event =

$$\frac{\text{odds of outcome event/odds of no event in control group}}{\text{odds of outcome event/odds of no outcome event in experimental group}}$$

$= (a/b)/(c/d)$
$= ad/bc$

For further examples of how to calculate the effects of therapy, see the excellent website http://www.eboncall.org/

Index

Note: page numbers in *italics* refer to figures and boxes, those in **bold** refer to tables.